THE LUMBAR SPINE

An atlas of normal anatomy
and the morbid anatomy of
ageing and injuries

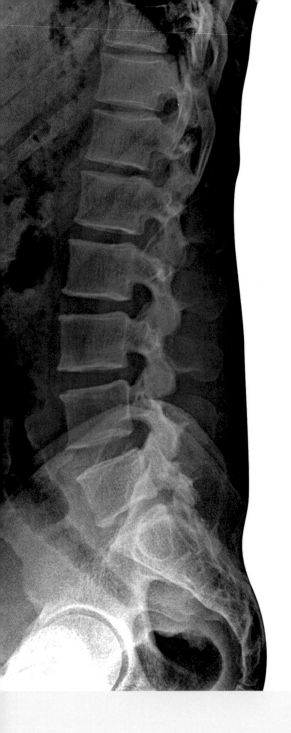

THE LUMBAR SPINE

An atlas of normal anatomy
and the morbid anatomy of
ageing and injuries

JAMES TAYLOR

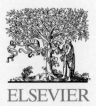

ELSEVIER

ELSEVIER

Elsevier Australia. ACN 001 002 357
(a division of Reed International Books Australia Pty Ltd)
Tower 2, 475 Victoria Avenue, Chatswood, NSW 2067

ISBN 978-0-7295-4313-2

Notice

Practitioners and researchers must always rely on their own experience and knowledge in evaluating and using any information, methods, compounds or experiments described herein. Because of rapid advances in the medical sciences, in particular, independent verification of diagnoses and drug dosages should be made. To the fullest extent of the law, no responsibility is assumed by Elsevier, authors, editors or contributors for any injury and/or damage to persons or property as a matter of product liability, negligence or otherwise, or from any use or operation of any methods, products, instructions or ideas contained in the material herein.

National Library of Australia Cataloguing-in-Publication Data

 A catalogue record for this book is available from the National Library of Australia

NATIONAL LIBRARY OF AUSTRALIA

Senior Content Strategist: Melinda McEvoy
Content Project Manager: Fariha Nadeem
Edited by Jo Crichton
Proofread by Annabel Adair
Cover and internal design by Georgette Hall
Typeset by GW Tech
Cover Image: Shutterstock/Xray computer (Image ID 450w-521571970)
Printed in Singapore by KHL Printing Co Pte Ltd

CONTENTS

FOREWORD

As an education and research-focused academic, I am frequently invited to review papers and book proposals. It is hard to express the excitement I felt when Professor Jim Taylor's *The Cervical Spine* draft came across my desk some years ago, followed a few years later by the draft of its companion, *The Lumbar Spine*. These atlases bring together the extensive, and arguably unmatched, research by Professor Taylor of the normal and morbid anatomy of the cervical and lumbar spine.

Professor James Taylor has a long and distinguished medical and academic career; his work on spinal anatomy is hard to match. Professor Taylor's work has informed and changed health professionals' understanding of anatomy and pathology of the spine. I first became aware of Professor Taylor's work in the mid-1990s when he published a series of articles on the cervical spine anatomy and morbidity. With each new publication, I, like many of my peers, paid attention.

As healthcare providers it is imperative that we understand both normal and pathological anatomy – it is often hard to find more than one example of pathology in a textbook. *The Lumbar Spine* provides unparalleled detail of normal, age-related changes and trauma-related injuries of the lumbar spine anatomy. All healthcare professionals with an interest in spinal health should be grateful that Professor Taylor has put these atlases together.

I have had the privilege of helping Professor Taylor to finalise both *The Cervical Spine* and *The Lumbar Spine* atlases. Working on these manuscripts was never a chore. Every clear and detailed image was a delight; every explanation provided me with further insights into the young, old and damaged human spine. As an undergraduate, I excelled at 'normal' anatomy. These books deepened my understanding of the normal, the ageing and the morbid human spine anatomy. I am honoured to have collaborated with Professor Taylor on this book and I commend it to all health professionals whose work involves the human spine.

Angie Fearon PhD, M (Phty), BAppSci (Phty), GCTE, FHEA, MAPA

PREFACE

This atlas presents pictures of normal, degenerate and injured lumbar spines, including bones, joints and muscles, garnered from studies of spinal autopsy specimens examined over a period of 33 years. They began with James Taylor's doctoral study at Edinburgh University, where he examined the developing spine (1967–74) and continued with studies of normal adult anatomy and age changes at the University of Western Australia (UWA), at Royal Perth Hospital (RPH) and in private practice (1976–2000).

Given careful observation, its 150 pictures and diagrams contain more information than many words could convey. Captions and labels have been kept to a minimum to avoid obscuring the images themselves. A short list of relevant literature is included in each section of the atlas.

THE MATERIAL STUDIED

Materials for study of the lumbar spine atlas have been collected since the 1960s. First, for the study of spinal development, and then for the study of normal anatomy, age changes and injuries, for which lumbar spine joints and whole lumbar spines were collected – both formalin-fixed material, and fresh, unfixed material. The latter were obtained both in the anatomy dissecting room and at autopsy in departments of pathology, to be examined at the request, or with the permission, of the pathologists.

To begin with, lumbar intervertebral discs and facet joints were embedded in cellulose or low-viscosity nitrocellulose and sectioned on a microtome (see Chapter 1 for methodology).

In later studies, whole unfixed lumbar spines were used for movement studies and formalin-fixed spines were studied for their normal anatomy or pathological features (see References for details).

The three doctoral studies making important contributions to this atlas are Giles (1987), Taylor (1974) and Twomey (1981).

Numerous articles describing the work have also appeared in peer-reviewed journals, books and book chapters. See, for example, McFadden and Taylor (1990), Taylor (1975), Taylor and Twomey (1980, 1986), Taylor, Twomey and Levander (2000), Twomey and Taylor (1982).

Further references are cited as appropriate.

ABOUT THE AUTHOR

James Taylor graduated MBChB at Edinburgh Medical School in 1955. He served as a GP surgeon in Congo as co-director of a hospital and medical training school founded by the late Sir Clement Chesterman, a Gallipoli veteran. In 1964 he returned to Edinburgh University to teach anatomy to medical students and undertake research on growth and development of the human spine, graduating with a PhD in 1974. Emigration to Australia in 1975 opened new research possibilities, including an attachment to the Sir George Bedbrook Spinal Unit at Royal Perth Hospital (RPH). Dr Taylor and his research team developed two new methods of sectioning autopsy spines. These methods (see Study Methods, page 2) gave high-quality and detailed information on the nature of blunt trauma injuries. As a consequence, he was invited to continue his spinal research in the Pathology Department at RPH, working with the forensic pathologists reporting to the coroner on blunt trauma spinal injuries in autopsy spines. This work provided access to study hundreds of spines from subjects of all ages.

Eminent spinal surgeons, radiologists and medical researchers, including Dr Nils Shonstrom and Professor Bo Levander from Sweden and Professor Ken McFadden from Canada, visited Dr Taylor for periods of cooperative research in his laboratory. On study leave, Dr Taylor continued to expand the range of his intervertebral disc research with Professsor John Scott, a world authority on proteoglycans.

In his last nine years before retirement, Dr Taylor was invited to work with Dr Philip Finch in his pain clinic. This work led to cooperative research of a clinical nature, particularly in the area of pain of spinal origin. Dr Finch, currently the Medical Director of Perth Pain Management Centre, has specialised in the field of pain medicine since 1978. Dr Finch gave the author invaluable help in the early stages of this atlas, reviewing the topic of disc innervation and discogenic pain.

Dr Taylor published an atlas on the cervical spine in 2019, which won first prize in the clinical science section of the Medical Book of the Year competition run by the British Medical Association in the United Kingdom.

ACKNOWLEDGEMENTS

There were many who contributed directly or indirectly to this book. The contributions of Mary Taylor and Mary Lee were essential in the processing, cutting and staining of 100-micron sections. Mary Taylor's part in the processing and photography of thick sections was equally important. Mary Taylor and Mary Lee also carefully measured the joint angles in a large number of CT scans. The radiologist, Dr Clem McCormick, worked with me comparing normal and abnormal CT scans with sections of cadaver spines. By inviting me to see spinal injury patients with chronic pain, Dr Philip Finch enabled me to compare autopsy injuries (e.g. 'rim lesions') with injuries (e.g. 'vacuum clefts') found in living patients. I am grateful to Dr Finch for his careful editing of the early chapters in this book.

I am grateful for the work and insights of my research colleagues from Australia and overseas. In particular, as the references cited indicate, research on age changes in the lumbar was done in close cooperation with Professor Lance Twomey. I am grateful to Lance for his fellowship and friendship over a period of 25 years of cooperative research and publications on the lumbar spine.

Thanks also to the staff at Elsevier for their patient help and sympathetic encouragement, especially during the COVID crisis.

Professor James Taylor MB, ChB, DTM, PhD, FAFRM (Sci)

April 2022

FIGURE REFERENCE GUIDE

The aims of the atlas are to:
- illustrate the functional anatomy of the normal lumbar spine based on examination of serial transverse and sagittal sections
- describe and illustrate age changes in the lumbar spine, showing how degenerative changes alter function and may cause pain and disability
- describe and portray the nature and distribution of lumbosacral spinal injuries due to blunt trauma, based on autopsy examinations of injured spines from blunt trauma deaths
- demonstrate to clinicians the areas vulnerable to injury.

THE AUTOPSY STUDIES

We present images of normal anatomy and the morbid anatomy of age changes and injuries. Our first studies were of sectioned lumbar facet joints; the embedding, sectioning at 100-micron thickness and staining were done in the Department of Anatomy and Human Biology at the University of Western Australia (UWA) by Mary Taylor and Mary Lee (Taylor & Twomey, 1986).

Serial sections of whole lumbar spines were made at Royal Perth Hospital (RPH) in the period from 1989 to June 1996 by James Taylor and Mary Taylor. Since then, a new coronial Act has restricted the possibility of examining parts of spines removed from cadavers.

Complete lumbar spines were examined as described below; the examinations were part of the forensic autopsies done routinely in the Department of Pathology at RPH where James Taylor and Mary Taylor assisted the forensic pathologists who had the responsibility of determining the cause of death in coroners' cases. Many spines were from young individuals who died from the effects of blunt trauma. We examined a large number of vertebrae and intervertebral joints showing normal anatomy and we were also able to research the nature of degenerative changes and spinal injuries (Taylor, Twomey & Levander, 2000).

Study methods

Two methods of sectioning were used. In the earlier study in the Department of Anatomy and Human Biology at UWA, individual spinal motion segments were decalcified, dehydrated, slowly embedded in low-viscosity nitrocellulose and sectioned at 100-micron thickness on a microtome. One in seven sections was stained with haematoxylin and light green colouring and mounted on a glass slide for microscopic examination. This method of preparation took about three months to complete. This method produced detailed histological information, but it was not capable of sectioning whole lumbar spines.

In the later study conducted in the Department of Pathology at RPH, whole lumbar spines of all ages were examined, from early childhood up to individuals over 80 years of age. The whole lumbar spine was expertly removed from the cadaver by a laboratory technician and fixed by immersion in formalin for 7 to 10 days, then embedded in 6.5% warm gelatin solution in a suitable container and deep frozen on dry ice at −70°C for 24–48 hours. The gelatin-enclosed frozen block was sectioned in 2.5 mm thick serial slices in the sagittal plane on a specially adapted band saw with a precision-adjustable guide and a fine-toothed blade (see Figure 1.1). The enclosure in gelatin before freezing allowed sectioning without damage to the surface of the spinal tissues as the blade passed smoothly from the frozen gelatin into the frozen spinal tissues. Cold burns while handling the block were avoided by wearing two pairs of rubber gloves.

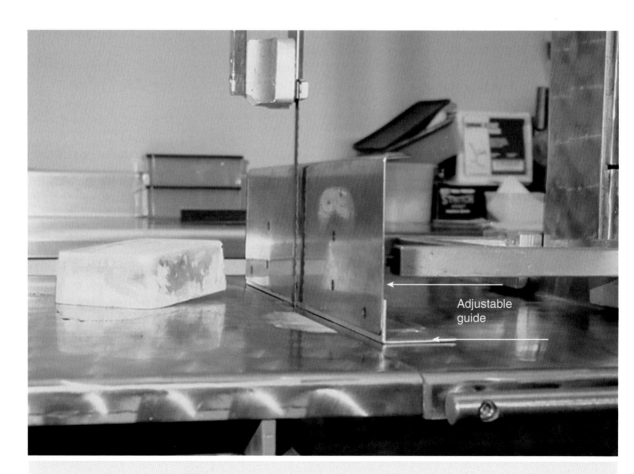

FIGURE 1.1 The modified band saw for sectioning spines

The saw table was fitted with a large, adjustable, precision guide (to regulate section thickness); a frozen block lies on the table, ready to be sectioned.

Each numbered slice was carefully washed and cleared of saw-cut debris and placed underwater in a large Petri dish to be photographed using a Pentax camera with a macro lens. Each slice was then examined under an M3 Leitz dissecting microscope at low magnification and closer pictures were taken of injuries or other structures of interest. Photography with the section underwater was necessary to avoid distortion by reflection of light from the surface of the section.

About 0.6 mm of tissue was lost as debris between successive sections. Sections were stored between numbered sheets of paper in 70% alcohol until the whole forensic examination of the case was complete. A written report on the nature and extent of injuries or other findings of interest was prepared for the forensic pathologist. This was included in the pathologist's report to the coroner to establish the cause of death (Taylor & Twomey, 1986).

FUNCTIONS OF THE LUMBAR SPINE

As a vital part of the axial skeleton, the lumbar spine's main functions are:
- stability in load-bearing
- movement
- protection of neural elements.

The human spine is uniquely adapted for erect posture, load-bearing and movement. It bears and transmits loads from the torso and upper limbs to the pelvis in an erect posture and in forward bending. The lumbar spine combines with hip joints and the thoracic spine to provide for movements required for bending, turning and reaching. The load-bearing function increases in a cranial to caudal direction, which is reflected in the progressive increase in area of the vertebral endplates from C3 to L3 or L4. The lumbar spine contains the lower end or conus of the spinal cord (at T12 to L1) with the central nervous centres for control of bowel and bladder function and lower limb reflexes. Below the cord, the lumbosacral spinal canal contains the cauda equina – the spinal nerves – which will supply the lower limbs.

The mechanical forces bearing on the lumbosacral spine throughout life may hasten the development of degenerative changes appearing in the bones (osteopenia and osteoporosis) and the joints (spondylosis), commencing in the intervertebral discs and then involving the facet joints.

This atlas will deal first with normal functional anatomy, then consider degenerative changes and the nature and consequences of injuries in the development of low back pain.

References

Taylor, JR & Twomey, LT 1986 Age changes in lumbar zygapophyseal joints. Observations on structure and function. *Spine*, 11(7), pp. 739–745.

Taylor, JL, Twomey, LT & Levander, B 2000 Contrasts between cervical and lumbar motion segments. *Critical Reviews in Physical and Rehabilitation Medicine*, 12(4), pp. 345–371.

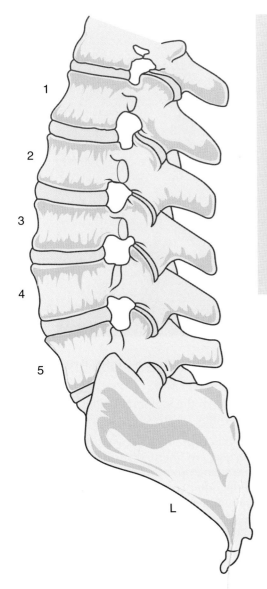

FIGURE 2.1 Sagittal view of the adult lumbar spine

The whole foetal vertebral column shows a 'primary' curve, concave anteriorly. The cervical spine develops a secondary curve convex forwards in infancy and the lumbar spine develops a lordotic posture in early childhood on adoption of the erect posture. The persisting primary curve of the thoracic spine shows a mild kyphosis. There are usually five lumbar vertebrae (occasionally 4 or 6 due to variation at the thoracic and sacral junctional areas). The lumbar lordosis is most marked in the lower lumbar segments and there is a sharp forward projecting angle at the lumbosacral junction. The sacrum is fused on each side with the ilia, transmitting loads through the pelvis to the lower limbs.

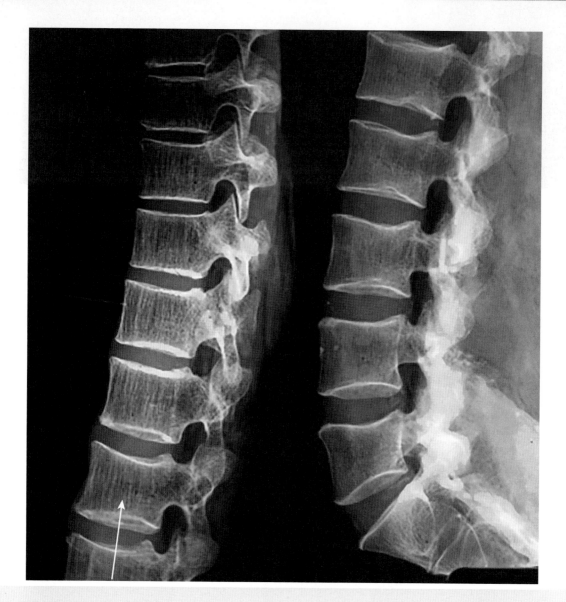

FIGURE 2.2 Normal lateral x-rays of thoracic (left) and lumbar spine (right) from a young adult cadaver

Note the predominantly vertical orientation of bony trabeculae in the vertebral bodies (arrow).

Each vertebral body has a thin outer shell of compact bone that contains a network of thin trabecular plates and spars of cancellous bone. Many trabeculae are oriented vertically to bear axial loads, but these are 'stiffened' by horizontal trabeculae to prevent them from bending to the point of fracture. The cancellous bone and the outer compact shell each bear about half of the axial load. The spaces within the bony honeycomb contain red marrow. Fibrocartilaginous intervertebral discs occupy the spaces between the vertebral bodies. The anterior height of L5 vertebral body is greater than its posterior height to accommodate the lumbosacral lordosis.

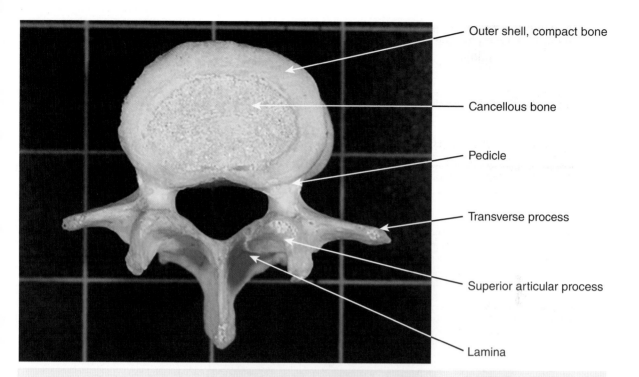

Outer shell, compact bone

Cancellous bone

Pedicle

Transverse process

Superior articular process

Lamina

FIGURE 2.3 A plan or axial view of an L3 lumbar vertebra

L3 has the longest transverse processes. It has a kidney-shaped vertebral body and a wide oval spinal canal. Note the medial-facing superior articular facets, with their posterior two-thirds in the sagittal plane and the anterior third curving medially towards the coronal plane. The rounded mammillary processes (for multifidus attachment) project back from the posterior extremity of each superior articular facet.

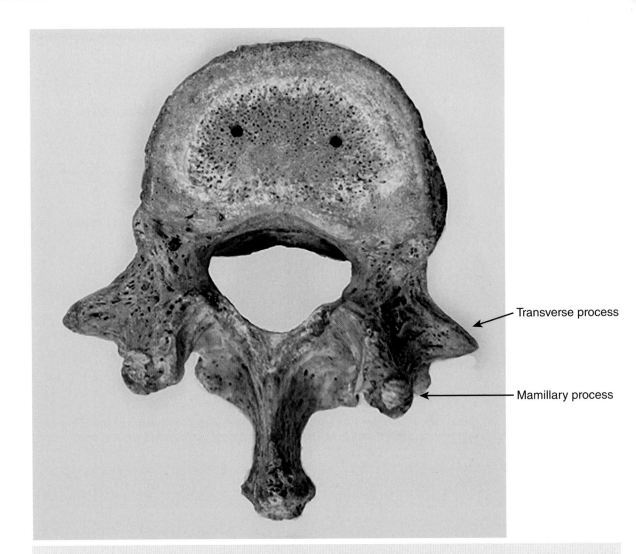

Transverse process

Mamillary process

FIGURE 2.4 A plan or axial view of an L5 vertebra

The vertebral body is rounded at the front and fairly flat at the back where the spinal canal is triangular in cross-section, with plenty of space laterally for the nerve roots.

L5 differs from the other lumbar vertebrae in having short stout 'conical' transverse processes which are attached to the iliac crest on each side by the ilio-lumbar ligaments. As this vertebra is angled forward in the lumbosacral spine in marked lordosis, part of the axial loading through the lumbosacral disc is shared by the L5 transverse processes and the ilio-lumbar ligament.

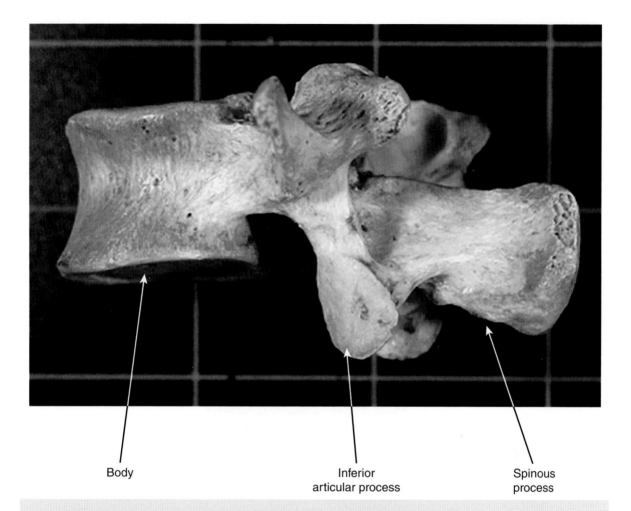

Body   Inferior   Spinous
         articular process   process

FIGURE 2.5 Lateral view of a normal lumbar vertebra

The vertebral endplates appear flat. The large, rectangular, spinous processes are described as 'hatchet-shaped'; the articular surface of the inferior articular process faces outward.

The strong pedicle passes back from the upper half of the vertebral body, leaving a deep notch below it for the exit passage of the spinal nerve through the upper part of the intervertebral foramen.

Partial ossification of ligamentum flavum

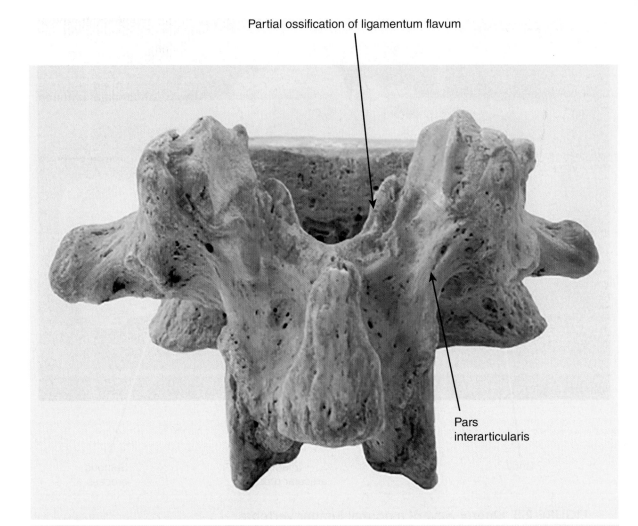

Pars
interarticularis

FIGURE 2.6 Posterior view of an individual lumbar vertebra

Between the four articular facets, the laminae cover and protect the spinal canal, enclosing the dural sac, which contains the cauda equina. The large spinous process projects back from the laminar junction in the midline. The elastic ligamentum flavum occupies the space between adjacent laminae; in this bone from an older subject, the ligament has been partly ossified.

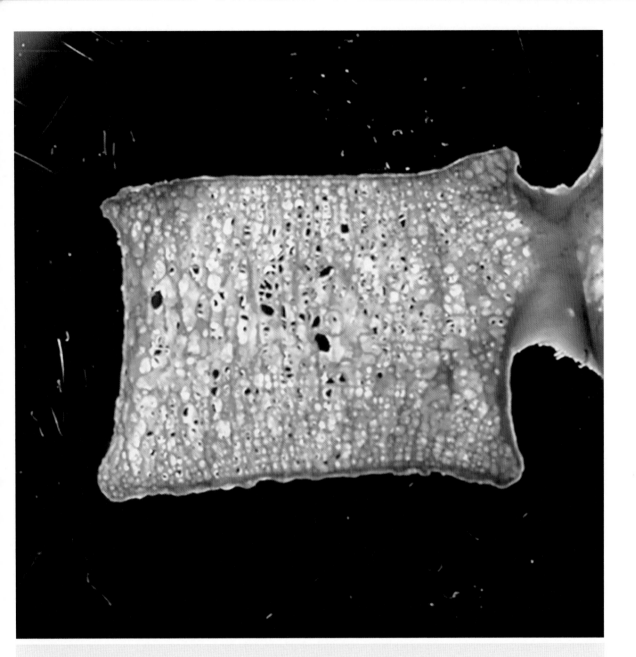

FIGURE 2.7 Sagittal section of vertebral body showing its inner structure

Vertically oriented trabeculae are supported by transverse ties which are more numerous near the vertebral endplates. Compare this with the x-rays in Figure 2.2, which show the vertical trabeculae well. The endplate is almost flat or slightly concave in a healthy vertebral body.

THE LUMBAR INTERVERTEBRAL JOINTS

1. The intervertebral disk

The fibrocartilaginous intervertebral discs are the strong load-bearing joints joining vertebral bodies.

2. The zygapophyseal joints (facet joints)

The zygapophyseal joints are the synovial joints between the vertebral arches. The facet joints are guide rails for intervertebral movements and they protect the discs from torsional or translational strain.

CHAPTER 3

INTERVERTEBRAL DISCS

The intervertebral disc has three parts:
- the nucleus pulposus
- the annulus fibrosus
- the cartilage plates.

The central nucleus pulposus is enclosed by the annulus fibrosus around its periphery and by the cartilage plates above and below. The cartilage plates are the unossified epiphyses of the vertebral body, but they are functionally part of the disc as they form the envelope enclosing the nucleus pulposus.

IMAGES OF DISCS IN TRANSVERSE SECTION

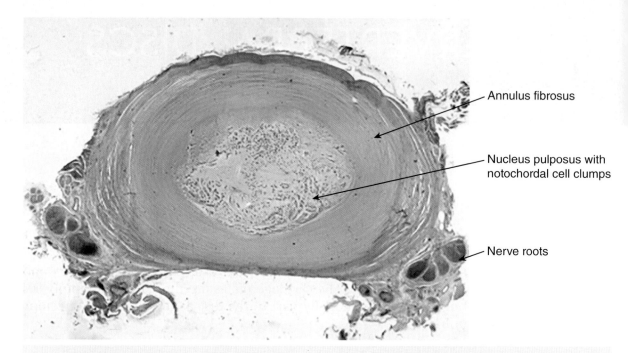

Annulus fibrosus

Nucleus pulposus with notochordal cell clumps

Nerve roots

FIGURE 3.1 The nucleus pulposus and annulus fibrosus in a stained, 100-micron transverse section of a full-term fetal lumbar disc

The annulus fibrosus encloses the fluid nucleus pulposus, which at this stage consists of notochordal cell clumps in a proteoglycan-rich matrix. The fetal nucleus is formed by the segmentation of the originally cylindrical notochord, with the extrusion of notochordal tissue from the rapidly growing vertebral bodies into the developing intervertebral discs. The annulus and the cartilage plates of the disc are vascular at this stage.

Anterior annulus fibrosus

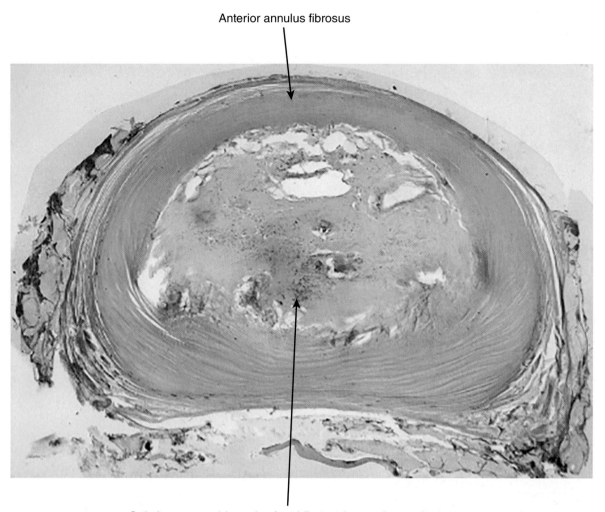

Gelatinous mucoid matrix of rapidly growing nucleus pulposus

FIGURE 3.2 Transverse 100-micron haematoxylin-stained section of a lumbar disc from a 3-year-old child

Note the large, expanded volume of the mucoid lumbar nucleus pulposus, which is much larger than a thoracic or cervical nucleus. The lamellar annulus of the child closely resembles that of a normal adult disc. The 'envelope' of the nucleus (annulus and cartilage plates) becomes avascular during childhood growth. The notochordal cells of the nucleus cannot survive in an avascular environment so they are replaced by fibroblasts with increased collagen formation.

The nucleus pulposus is a fluid structure in infancy and childhood, becoming less fluid but still capable of deformation in adolescents and young adults. According to Nachemson and Elfstrom (1970), it still behaves like a fluid in adults, although with advancing age its collagen content continues to increase, and it becomes less capable of herniation through a ruptured annulus.

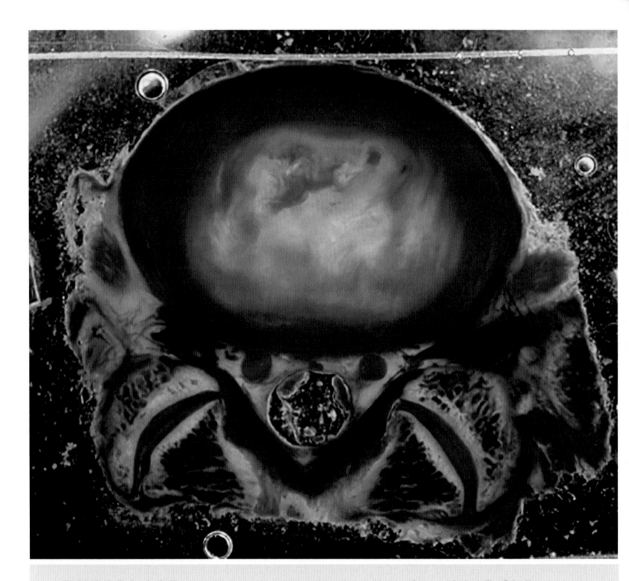

FIGURE 3.3 A 2.5 mm transverse unstained section of an adult L5–S1 disc

With dark-ground illumination, the annulus appears dark orange. The large central nucleus pulposus of the adult has a high water content and is rich in proteoglycans. It is enclosed by the annulus fibrosus around its periphery and by the cartilage plates above and below. The antero-lateral annulus is thicker than the posterior annulus. The facet joints and local spinal nerves are also shown.

IMAGES OF DISCS IN SAGITTAL SECTION

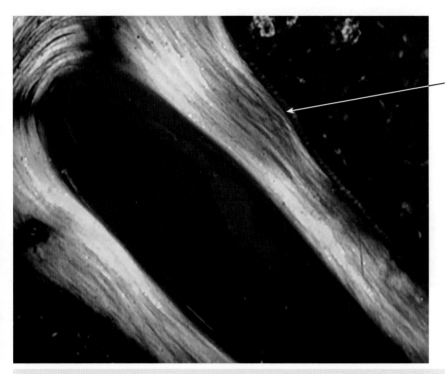

Lamellar arrangement of cartilage plate corresponds with the lamellar arrangement of the annulus fibrosus.

FIGURE 3.4 A child's lumbar disc viewed by polarised light

A child's lumbar disc viewed by polarised light (Taylor, 1975) shows the continuity of the lamellar annulus with the lamellar structure of the cartilage endplate.

Note the lamellar structure of both annulus and cartilage plate.

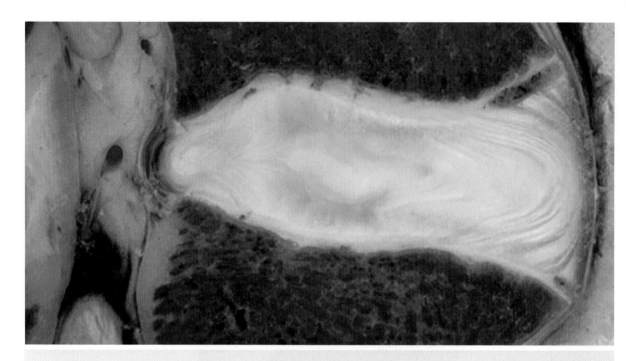

FIGURE 3.5 Sagittal section of a young adult lumbar intervertebral disc

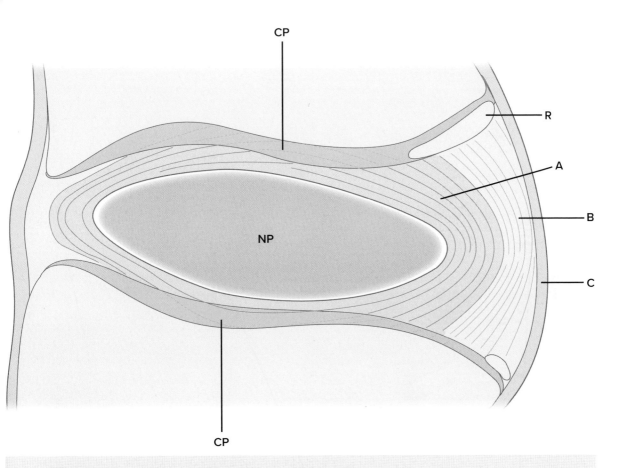

CP

R

A

B

C

NP

CP

FIGURE 3.6 A diagrammatic copy of Figure 3.5

This shows the anterior longitudinal ligament covering the anterior annulus and demonstrates the different parts of the anterior annulus and the cartilage plates.

The anterior annulus (B) is covered by the anterior longitudinal ligament (C). The outer annulus (B) attaches to the ring apophysis (R), which fuses with the vertebral body, at skeletal maturity, as the vertebral rim. The inner lamellae of the annulus (A) are in direct continuity with lamellae in the cartilage plates (CP). NP = nucleus pulposus.

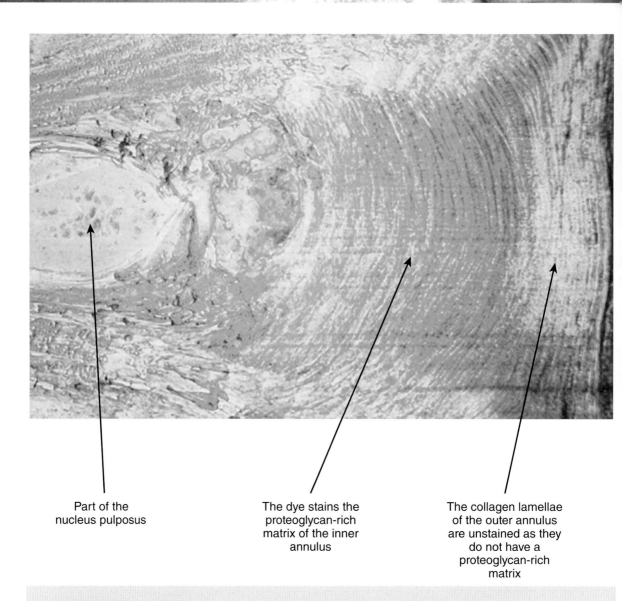

Part of the
nucleus pulposus

The dye stains the
proteoglycan-rich
matrix of the inner
annulus

The collagen lamellae
of the outer annulus
are unstained as they
do not have a
proteoglycan-rich
matrix

FIGURE 3.7 A 100-micron section shows alcian blue staining of the inner annulus of a child

Taylor et al., 1992

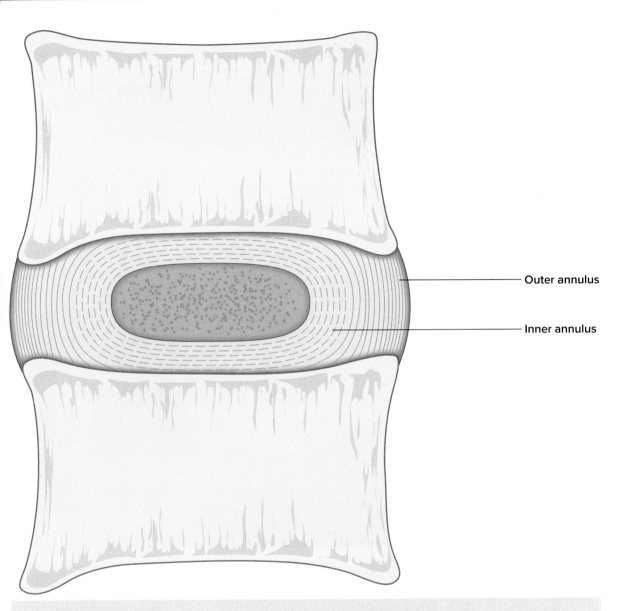

Outer annulus

Inner annulus

FIGURE 3.8 Diagram of an adult lumbar disc in mid-sagittal section

The continuous lamellae of the inner fibrocartilaginous annulus and cartilage plates form an envelope enclosing the nucleus pulposus; the outer collagenous annulus simply bridges between the outer vertebral rims above and below.

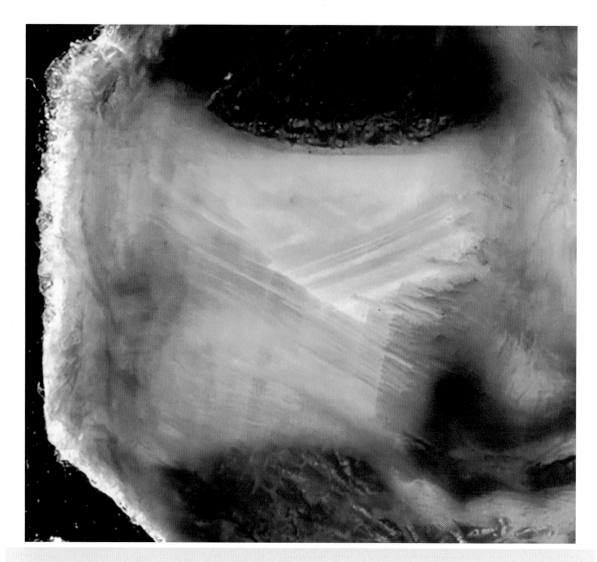

FIGURE 3.9 A 2.5 mm thick sagittal section of the outer annulus

This figure shows the alternating direction of the fibres in adjacent lamellae with an interstriation angle of about 50°. There are about 15 or 16 concentric collagenous lamellae in the annulus; adjacent layers pass in contrasting directions to give added strength to the disc.

Descriptions of discs as constructed by an annulus and a nucleus are no longer adequate. The outer annulus (as previously described) bridges the gap from vertebral body to vertebral body. The continuity of the inner annulus, with the cartilage plates above and below, give it a different function compared with the outer annulus. This conclusion is reinforced by their different staining characteristics; the collagenous outer annulus has a low proteoglycan content; the inner annulus and the cartilage plates are rich in proteoglycans, reflecting an axial load-bearing function.

In this figure, the outer lamellae bind the two adjacent vertebral bodies together and resist or control hyperextension, hyperflexion and axial rotation.

THE CARTILAGE ENDPLATES

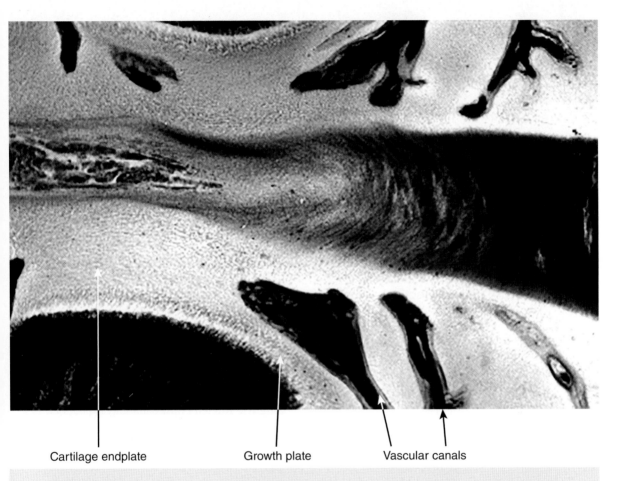

Cartilage endplate   Growth plate   Vascular canals

FIGURE 3.10 A coronal section of the right half of a young child's lumbar disc

This coronal section of a young child's lumbar disc shows vascular canals in the cartilage plates approaching the nucleus pulposus and the inner annulus. The vascular canals end in capillary networks close to the disc. The cartilage plates are vascular in infants and children but avascular in adults. The darker part of the cartilage plate adjoining the vertebral body is its growth plate.

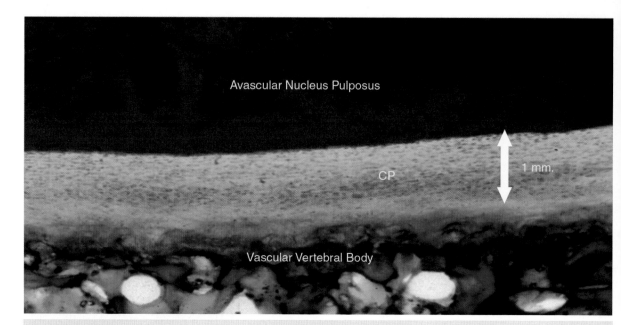

FIGURE 3.11 Sagittal section of the cartilage plate from a young adult

The human hyaline cartilage endplate (CP) is stained by haematoxylin and light green.

The human hyaline cartilage plate is the unossified epiphysis of the vertebral body. It is only around its periphery that a bony ring appears at adolescence to fuse with the vertebral body as the vertebral rim. This contrasts sharply with the bony plate epiphysis of quadrupedal mammals.

The CP is an essential part of the 'envelope' enclosing the nucleus pulposus and it is also a principal pathway for diffusion of oxygen and glucose to the adult avascular disc from the vascular vertebral body, via small vascular buds. It is intimately attached to the inner annulus, and both structures form the inner envelope enclosing the nucleus pulposus.

DISC NUTRITION

The intervertebral disc is highly vascular during the rapid growth period in infancy and early childhood, but during childhood growth, blood vessels disappear from the cartilage plates and annulus (Taylor et al., 2000). Disc nutrition in the adult depends on diffusion of oxygen and nutrients from vascular buds at the bone-cartilage plates' interface and from the small blood vessels on the surface of the disc into the large fibro-cartilaginous disc. Adequate diffusion of the nutrients and oxygen through the disc tissues is in part dependent on regular movement (Grunhagen et al., 2011; Urban et al., 2004).

The component tissues of the intervertebral disc include collagen and proteoglycans. Collagen predominates in the outer annulus, but the inner annulus and nucleus pulposus each have a matrix rich in proteoglycans. The proteoglycan-rich central tissues of the disc are related to their load-bearing functions as they could attract more water than their enclosure by the outer annulus and cartilage plates will allow. When the fresh post-mortem disc is sectioned, its centre swells and buckles as the proteoglycans of the nucleus and inner annulus absorb water from the atmosphere.

The outward pressure of the disc centre and inner annulus balances the external, compressive axial load. During daytime activity, each disc is slightly compressed by the squeezing-out of water. This daily 'creep' makes an individual up to an inch shorter in stature by the evening. During the night, in recumbent posture, the disc reabsorbs water and the individual recovers maximum stature.

Twomey and Taylor (1982) showed that from the end of normal flexion, prolonged loading for one hour produced further flexion due to 'creep'. On releasing the external loading, the spine gradually reversed the creep (hysteresis) due to the reestablishment of water within the disc as determined by its proteoglycan content and distribution.

LOAD-BEARING AND MOVEMENT

Load-bearing occurs predominantly through the vertebral bodies and intervertebral discs. The discs have a limited capacity to deform in movement and the types and ranges of movement (for example, in the sagittal and axial planes) are controlled by facet orientation.

The intervertebral discs transmit axial loads. The annulus is described as the principal load-bearing structure (Lundon & Bolton, 2001) or, to be more precise, the inner ring of the annulus and the cartilage plates, which enclose the nucleus pulposus, bear the load. This load-bearing by the annulus (Lundon & Bolton, 2001) is supported by the structure and chemistry of the disc, especially its proteoglycan content, which attracts water into the disc. The nucleus itself, behaving as a fluid, acts as a shock-absorbing mechanism when subject to sudden increases in loading (David et al., 2000). The nucleus can redistribute axial loads centripetally.

Discs can change shape allowing movement in the sagittal, transverse and axial planes. The collagenous structure of the outer annulus, principally type-1 collagen, is adapted to perform a stabilising and restraining mechanism at the limits of normal movement. The orientation of the facets is also adapted to prevent excessive sagittal-plane or axial-twisting movements, which may damage the annulus.

References

David, W, Huki, N & Meakin, JR 2000 Relationship between structure and mechanical function of the tissues of the intervertebral joint. *American Zoologist*, 40(1), pp. 42–52.

Grunhagen, T, Shirazi-Adl, A, Fairbank, JC & Urban, JP 2011 Intervertebral disk nutrition: a review of factors influencing concentrations of nutrients and metabolites. *Orthopedic Clinics of North America*, 42(4), pp. 465–477, vii.

Lundon, K & Bolton, K 2001 Structure and function of the lumbar intervertebral disk in health, aging, and pathologic conditions. *Journal of Orthopaedic & Sports Physical Therapy*, 31(6), pp. 291–303; discussion pp. 304–296.

Nachemson, A & Elfstrom, G 1970 Intravital dynamic pressure measurements in lumbar discs. A study of common movements, maneuvers and exercises. *Scandinavian Journal of Rehabilitation Medicine Supplement*, 1, pp. 1–40.

Taylor, JR 1975 Growth of human intervertebral discs and vertebral bodies. *Journal of Anatomy*, 120(1), pp. 49–68.

Taylor, JR, Scott, JE, Cribb, AM & Bosworth, TR 1992 Human intervertebral disc acid glycosaminoglycans. *Journal of Anatomy*, 180(1), pp. 137–141.

Taylor, JL, Twomey, LT & Levander, B 2000 Contrasts between cervical and lumbar motion segments. *Critical Reviews in Physical and Rehabilitation Medicine*, 12(4), pp. 345–371.

Twomey, L & Taylor, J 1982 Flexion creep deformation and hysteresis in the lumbar vertebral column. *Spine*, 7(2), pp. 116–122.

Urban, JP, Smith, S & Fairbank, JC 2004 Nutrition of the intervertebral disc. *Spine*, 29(23), pp. 2700–2709.

Further reading

Maroudas, A, Stockwell, RA, Nachemson, A & Urban, J 1975 Factors involved in the nutrition of the human lumbar intervertebral disc: cellularity and diffusion of glucose in vitro. *Journal of Anatomy*, 120(1), pp. 113–130.

Scott, JE, Bosworth, TR, Cribb, AM & Taylor, JR 1994 The chemical morphology of age-related changes in human intervertebral disc glycosaminoglycans from cervical, thoracic and lumbar nucleus pulposus and annulus fibrosus. *Journal of Anatomy*, 184(1), pp. 73–82.

Taylor, JR & Twomey, LT 1979 Innervation of lumbar intervertebral discs. *Medical Journal of Australia*, 2(13), pp. 701–702.

Taylor, J & Twomey, L 1980 Innervation of lumbar intervertebral discs. *New Zealand Journal of Physiotherapy*, 8, pp. 36–37.

CHAPTER 4

THE ZYGAPOPHYSEAL JOINTS

The zygapophyseal or facet joints are the synovial joints between vertebral arches. They act as guide rails, facilitating intervertebral movements in the sagittal and coronal planes but limiting axial rotation and anterior translation, protecting the discs from shearing and twisting.

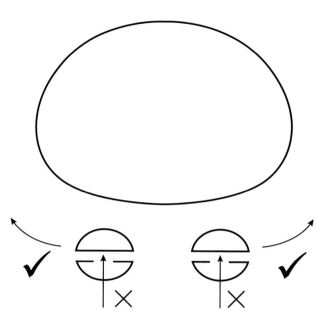

1. Coronal orientation prevents forward TRANSLATION, favours AXIAL ROTATION.

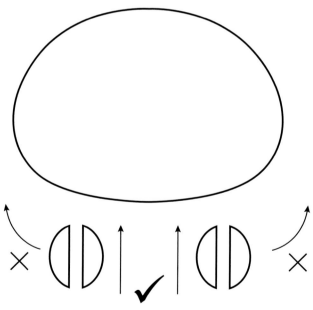

2. Sagittal orientation allows forward TRANSLATION, but resists AXIAL ROTATION.

FIGURES 4.1 AND 4.2 Facet orientation

The facet orientation protects the discs from inappropriate movements. Biplanar orientation protects the disc from anterior translation and torsional shear.

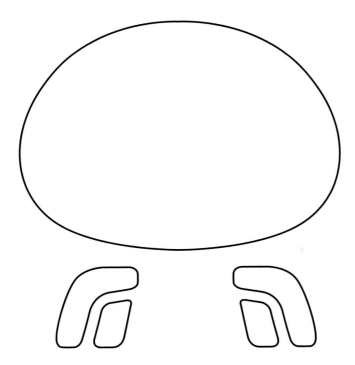

3. Biplanar orientation limits BOTH forward **TRANSLATION**,
and **AXIAL ROTATION** and protects the i.v. discs from
both **TWISTING** and **SHEARING** forces.

FIGURE 4.3 Facet orientation

The superior articular facets in a foetus and infant are oriented entirely in the coronal
plane. The sagittally oriented parts grow backwards in a child in response to load-bearing,
to achieve the 'biplanar' orientation of the adult, as shown above.

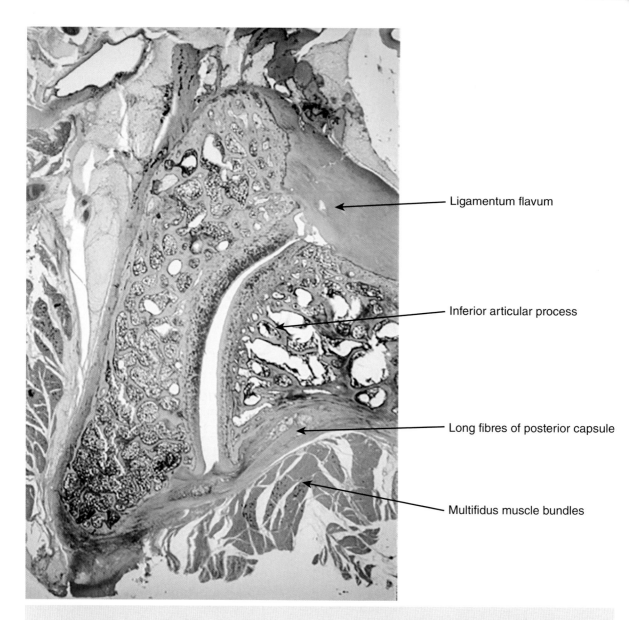

Ligamentum flavum

Inferior articular process

Long fibres of posterior capsule

Multifidus muscle bundles

FIGURE 4.4 A 100-micron stained transverse section of an L3–4 facet joint from a young female adult

The posterior two-thirds of the joint are in the sagittal plane and its anterior third is curving round towards the coronal plane. The joint is enclosed anteriorly by the elastic ligamentum flavum and posteriorly by a fibrous capsule, part of which attaches to the inferior facet some distance medial to the joint. The articular processes are covered laterally and posteriorly by fibres of the multifidus muscle.

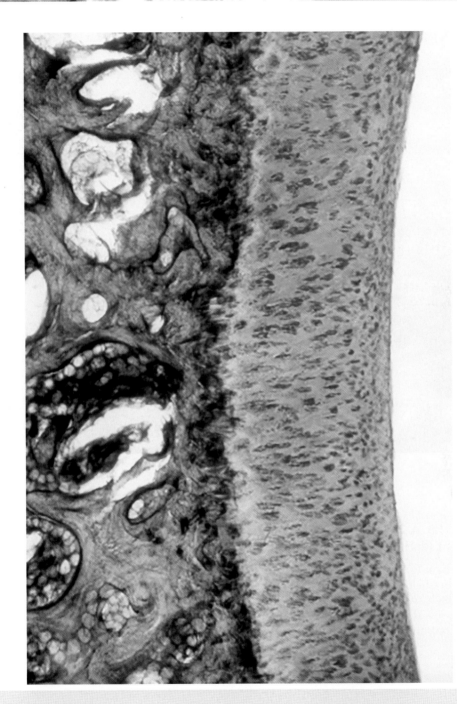

FIGURE 4.5 A higher-power view of the articular cartilage and part of its sub-chondral bone plate

There are plentiful chondrocytes and a very smooth articular surface. The collagen content of the cartilage is not shown, but its orientation perpendicular to the bone plate is suggested by the orientation of the oval chondrocytes.

Superior articular facet

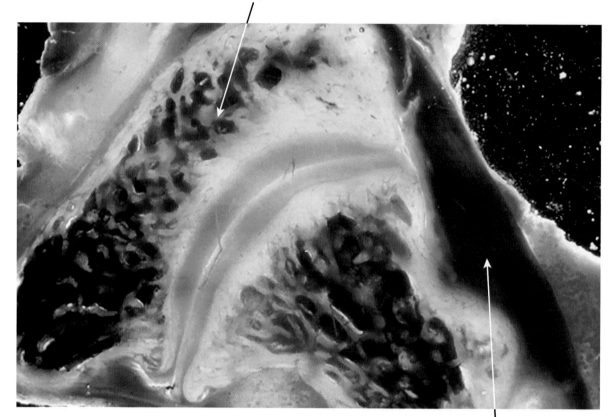

Ligamentum flavum

FIGURE 4.6 A 2.5 mm thick, unstained transverse section of a normal lumbar facet joint (dark-ground illumination)

The convex inferior articular facet fits closely into the concave superior articular facet of the vertebra below. The articular cartilages are supported by dense sub-chondral bone plates, which are thicker anteriorly due to greater loading of this part. The ligamentum flavum forms the anterior capsule of the joint and also joins adjacent laminae, giving a smooth continuous surface for the dural sac and its contents.

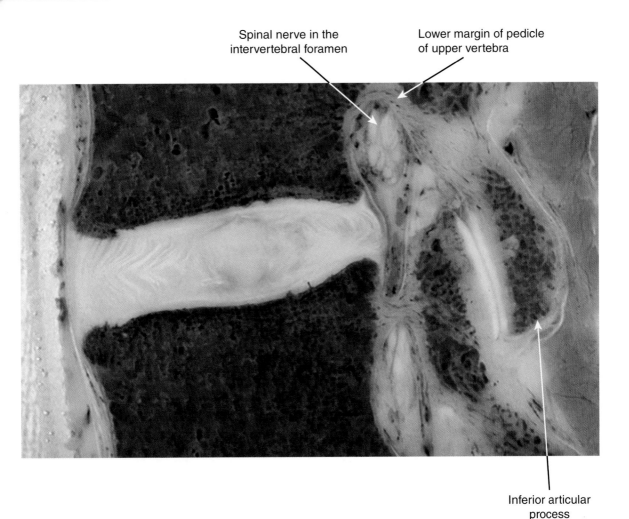

Spinal nerve in the intervertebral foramen

Lower margin of pedicle of upper vertebra

Inferior articular process

FIGURE 4.7 A parasagittal section through the disc, pedicle and facet joint

The inferior articular process of the upper vertebra projects almost vertically downwards, like a 'hook', behind the superior articular process of the next vertebra.

This prevents excessive forward translation of the upper vertebra on the lower vertebra in flexion with consequent shearing forces in the disc. There is a slight forward slope in the lumbar facet joint surfaces, averaging about 8°. This increases from above, downwards from L1 to L5. This slope allows about 2–3 mm of translation to accompany full forward rotation in flexion (Kozanek et al., 2009; Taylor & Twomey, 1986).

AVERAGE JOINT PLANE

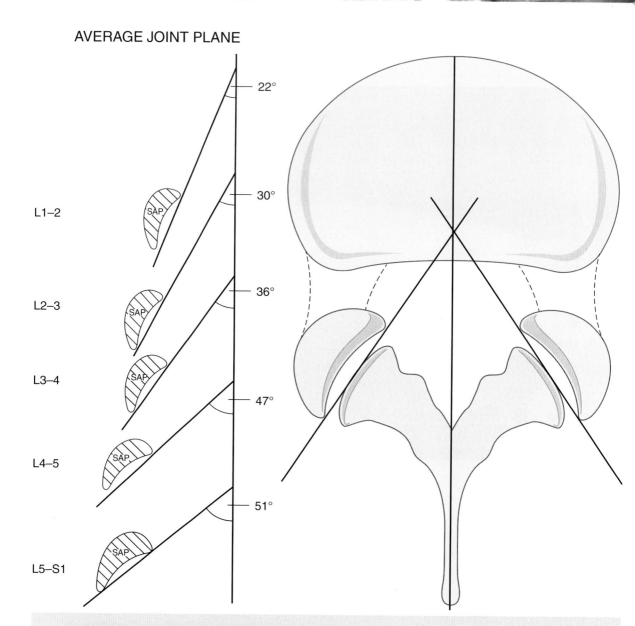

FIGURE 4.8 Increasing lordosis from above down in the lumbar spine is accompanied by increase in the joint angle

The increasing lordosis is associated with increased loading of the lower facet joints. Measurement of the 'facet angle' in the axial plane was performed in up to 200 CT scans; the average angle at each level is shown. The largest intersegmental increase is from L3–4 to L4–5. SAP: superior articular process.

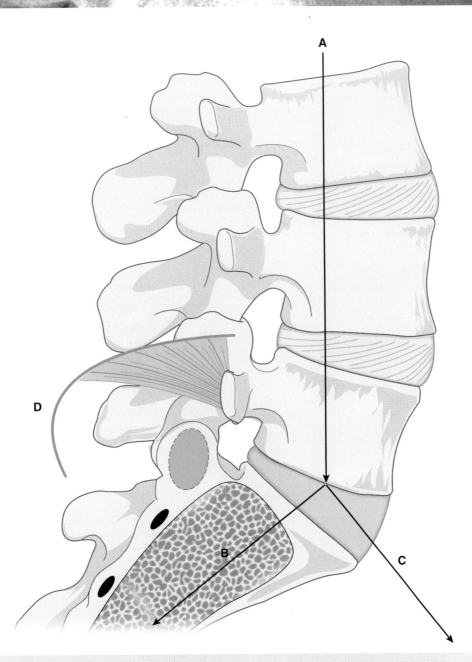

FIGURE 4.9 The lumbosacral joints showing the division of forces

Most axial loading passes through the vertebral bodies and intervertebral discs, but the proportion of the load borne by the facets in erect posture and forward flexion increases at the hyper-lordotic lower levels. With increasing lordosis at L4–5 and L5–S1, there is a progressive increase in loading of the facets and of shearing forces in the disc.

These shearing forces (C) are resisted by:

1. the lumbosacral facet joints (blue)
2. the ilio-lumbar ligaments (green D).

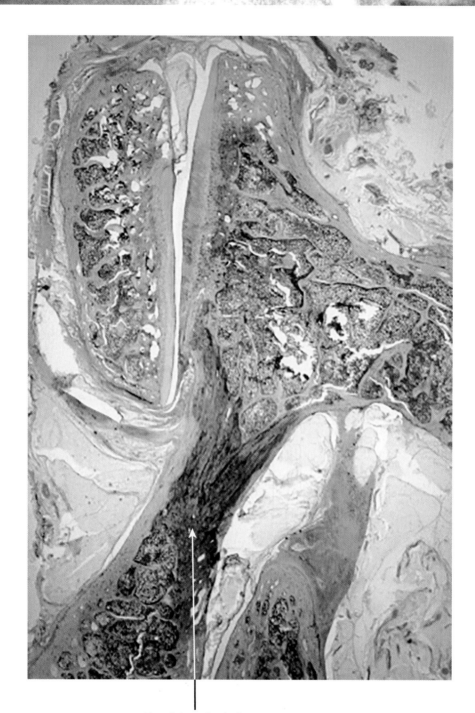

Pars interarticularis

FIGURE 4.10 The pars interarticularis

A 100-micron stained sagittal section of a lower lumbar pars interarticularis. Loading of this structure causes a dense bone response with increased staining. The pars interarticularis in lower lumbar vertebrae endures significant loading in movements (Taylor & McCormick, 1991).

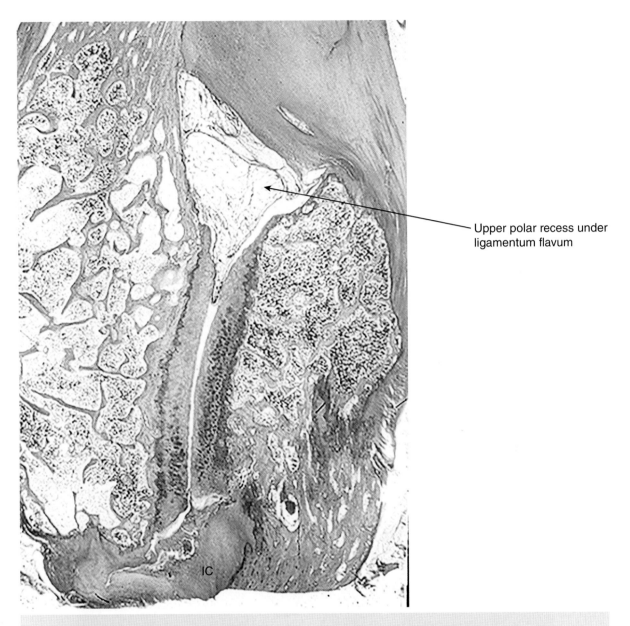

Upper polar recess under ligamentum flavum

IC

FIGURE 4.11 Polar recesses of lumbar facet joints in sagittal section

The polar recesses of the facet joints accommodate flexion and extension movements in the sagittal plane. The recesses contain fat pads lined by synovial membrane.

The inferior capsule (IC) shows abnormal thickening.

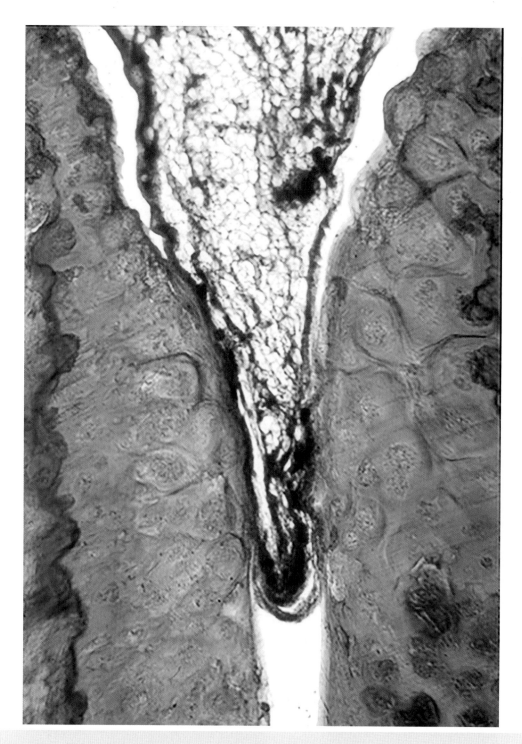

FIGURE 4.12 Fat-filled, facet joint vascular synovial folds

Fat-filled, vascular synovial folds project from the polar recesses between the articular surfaces. These synovial folds move freely in and out of the joints during movement.

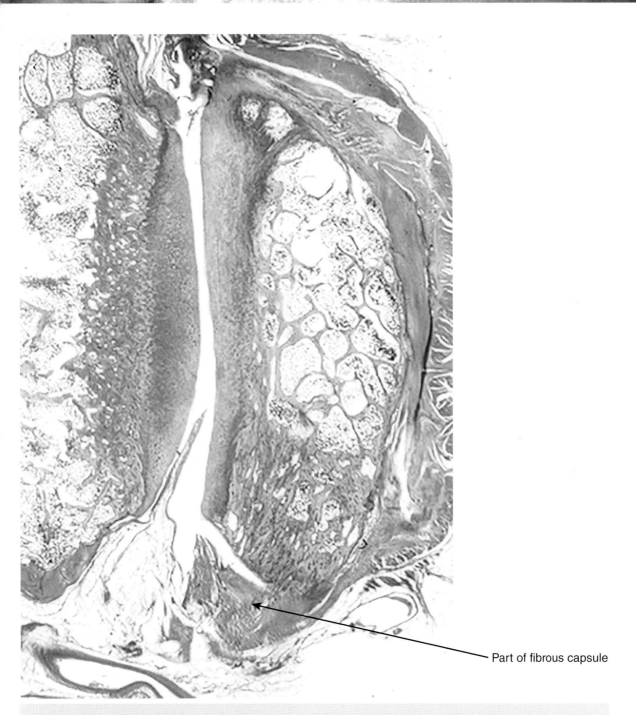

Part of fibrous capsule

FIGURE 4.13 Extra-articular fat pads

Extra-articular fat pads lie in bony hollows on the laminae below the lower lumbar facet joints and connect with the lower intra-articular synovial folds through a hole in the lower capsule. The fat pads accommodate downward movements of the facet in full extension.

References

Kozanek, M, Wang, S, Passias, PG et al. 2009 Range of motion and orientation of the lumbar facet joints in vivo. *Spine*, 34(19), pp. E689–696.

Taylor, JR & McCormick, CC 1991 Lumbar facet joint fat pads: their normal anatomy and their appearance when enlarged. *Neuroradiology*, 33(1), pp. 38–42.

Taylor, JR & Twomey, LT 1986 Age changes in lumbar zygapophyseal joints. Observations on structure and function. *Spine*, 11(7), pp. 739–745.

Further reading

Giles, LG 1987 The anatomy of lower lumbar and lumbosacral joint recesses with particular reference to their innervation. University of Western Australia, Perth.

Giles, LG & Taylor, JR 1987 Human zygapophyseal joint capsule and synovial fold innervation. *British Journal of Rheumatology*, 26(2), pp. 93–98.

Giles, LG, Taylor, JR & Cockson, A 1986 Human zygapophyseal joint synovial folds. *Acta Anatomica* (Basel), 126(2), pp. 110–114.

Pearcy, MJ & Tibrewal, SB 1984 Axial rotation and lateral bending in the normal lumbar spine measured by three-dimensional radiography. *Spine*, 9(6), pp. 582–587.

Taylor, J & Twomey, L 1980 Sagittal and horizontal plane movement of the human lumbar vertebral column in cadavers and in the living. *Rheumatology and Rehabilitation*, 19(4), pp. 223–232.

Twomey, L, Taylor, J & Furniss, B 1983 Age changes in the bone density and structure of the lumbar vertebral column. *Journal of Anatomy*, 136(1), pp. 15–25.

Taylor, J, Twomey, L & Levander, B 2000 Contrasts between cervical and lumbar motion segments. *Critical Reviews in Physical and Rehabilitation Medicine*, 12(4), pp. 345–371.

CHAPTER 5

LUMBAR SPINAL NERVES

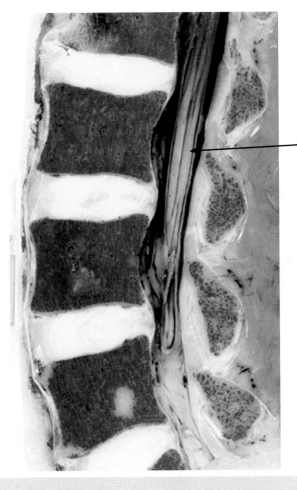

Cauda equina in dural sac

FIGURE 5.1 The cauda equina in mid-sagittal section

This thick sagittal section of lumbar spine shows the cauda equina in the dural sac.

The cord terminates at L1–2.

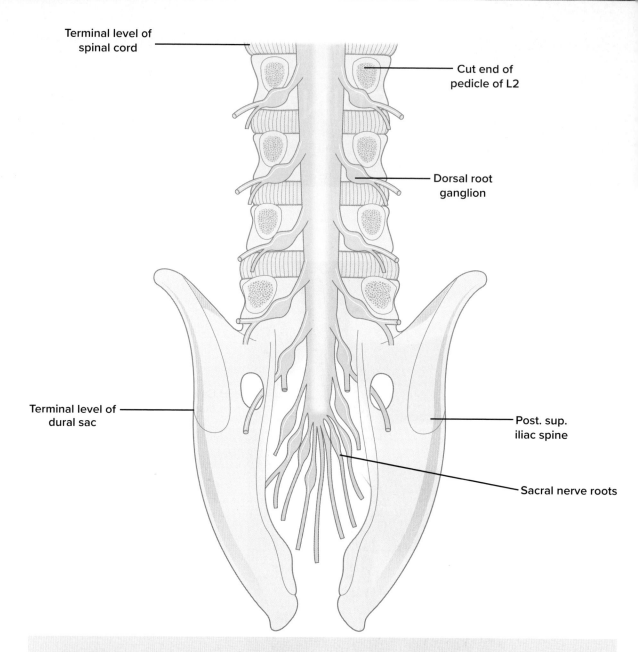

Terminal level of
spinal cord

Cut end of
pedicle of L2

Dorsal root
ganglion

Terminal level of
dural sac

Post. sup.
iliac spine

Sacral nerve roots

FIGURE 5.2 The lumbosacral dural sac

Diagram of the lumbosacral part of the dural sac, viewed from behind, showing the origin of the spinal nerves in their dural sleeves. The cauda equina are bathed in cerebrospinal fluid (CSF) within the sac. As the spinal nerves leave the dural sac to pass inferiorly to the pedicles, they are covered by a dural sleeve containing CSF.

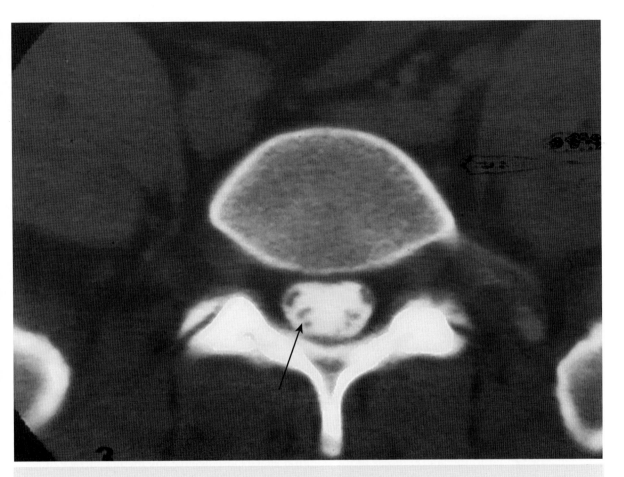

FIGURE 5.3 Cauda equina in an axial CT section of lumbar spine

Cauda equina in the dural sac are outlined by radiological contrast agent.

The cauda equina are 'lined up' in series (see arrow). The lumbar CT-myelogram shows the cauda equina as negative images in white contrast material.

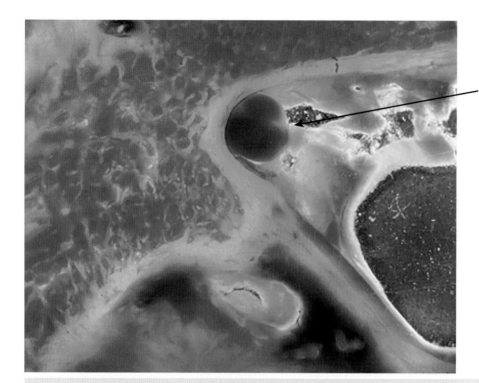

Nerve roots in the lateral recess of the spinal canal

FIGURE 5.4 Nerve roots in the lateral recess

A thick unstained transverse section of the left half of the spinal canal.

The large dorsal nerve root and the small motor root in front of it (dark brown) are enclosed in fat in the lateral recess of the epidural space close against the medial surface of the pedicle.

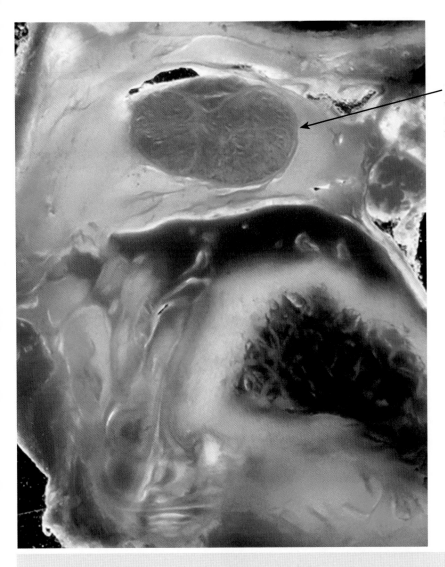

Dorsal root ganglion fusing with small flat anterior motor root in the upper intervertebral foramen

FIGURE 5.5 Spinal nerve roots

A thick transverse section shows the spinal nerve roots, enclosed in fat. The small anterior motor root joins the dorsal root ganglion in the upper intervertebral foramen as they exit the spinal canal.

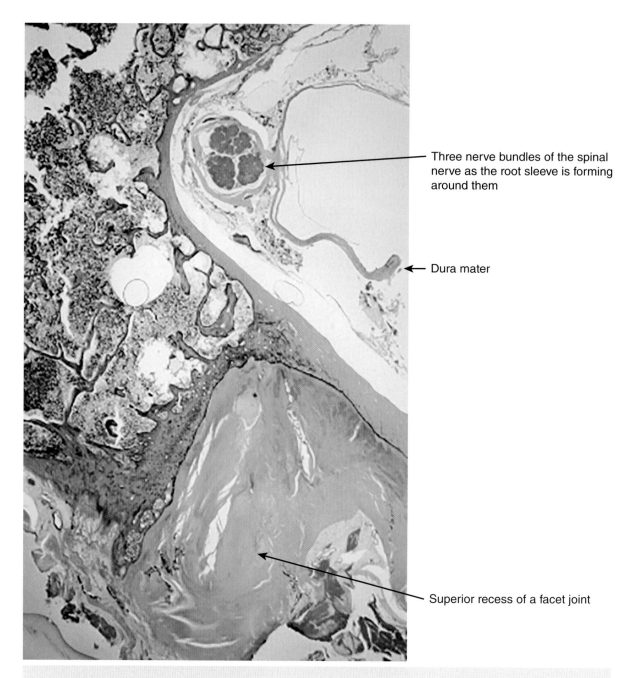

Three nerve bundles of the spinal nerve as the root sleeve is forming around them

Dura mater

Superior recess of a facet joint

FIGURE 5.6 Spinal nerve in the spinal canal lateral recess

A 100-micron stained transverse section shows a spinal nerve in the lateral recess of the spinal canal at L3–4. The root sleeve is budding off the dural sac.

Pedicle

Posterior margin of vertebral body

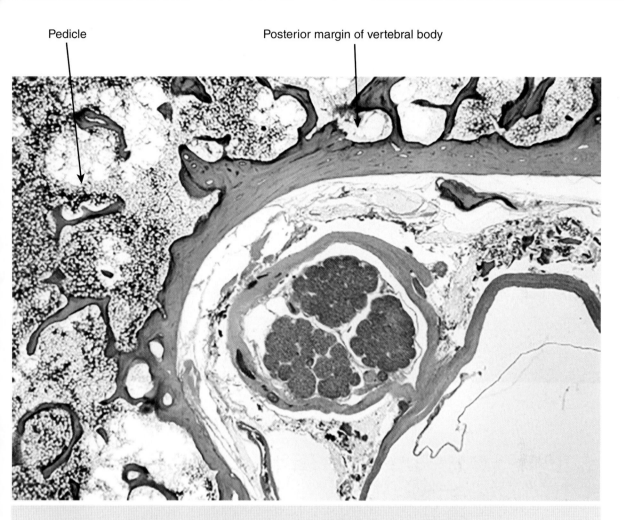

FIGURE 5.7 Higher-power view of the formation of the root sleeve

This section shows a higher-power view of the formation of the root sleeve around the nerve root. Three fascicles of the nerve root are visible.

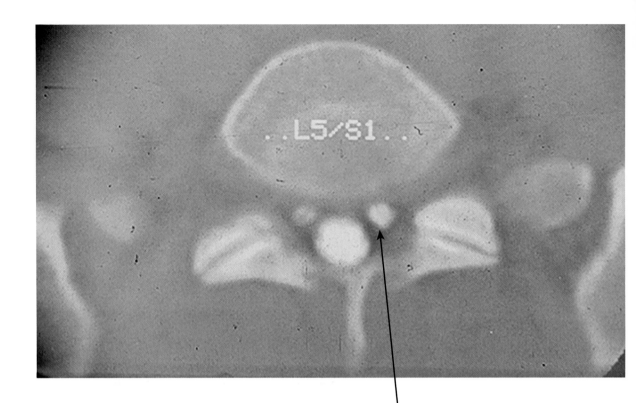

Contrast has spread into root sleeve

FIGURE 5.8 An axial CT myelogram at L5–S1

A CT myelogram of a normal young adult shows the spread of contrast from the dural sac into the root sleeves.

The root sleeve is seen
enclosing the nerve
roots

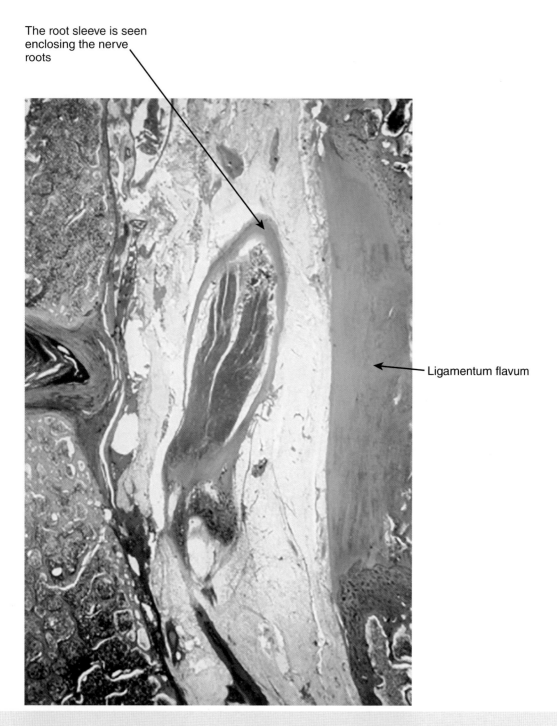

Ligamentum flavum

FIGURE 5.9 A para-sagittal section of the lumbar spinal canal

The thick dorsal root and the thin ventral nerve root descend within their root sleeve
towards their exit at the intervertebral foramen. Part of the posterior disc is seen in front
of the canal.

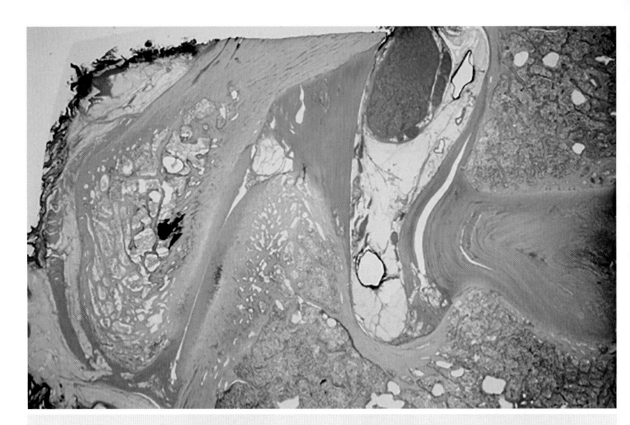

FIGURE 5.10 A 100-micron stained sagittal section of the intervertebral foramen with the nerve roots in the upper foramen

The dorsal root ganglion and the small, flat motor root are in the upper foramen accompanied by a vein. A second vein is at disc level in the lower foramen. The ligamentum flavum forms the posterior boundary of the canal.

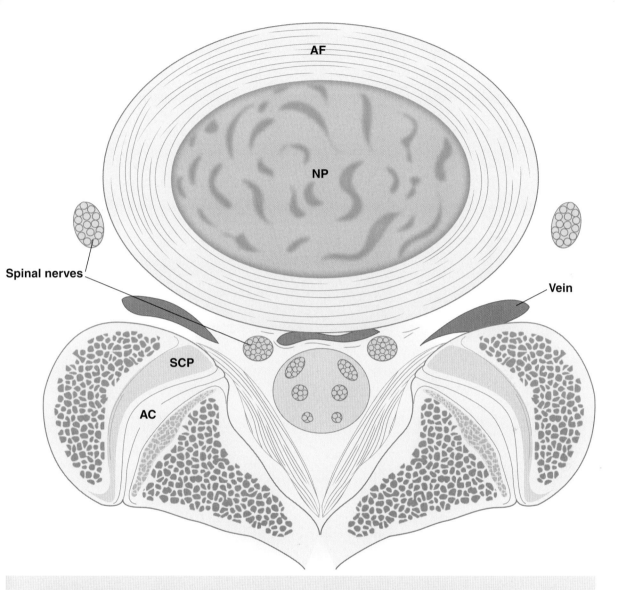

FIGURE 5.11 The close relations of spinal nerves to the L5–S1 disc

The close relations of spinal nerves to the L5–S1 disc are shown in a tracing of a thick unstained transverse section (see Figure 5.3). In the spinal canal, the S1 spinal nerves lie in contact with the posterior surface of the disc and the L5 nerves lie close to the postero-lateral surface of the disc. Other sacral nerves are still within the lower dural sac.

(AC = articular cartilage, AF = annular fibrosis, NP = nucleus pulposus, SCP = subchondral bone plate)

CHAPTER 6

VESSELS OF THE SPINAL CANAL

Anterior spinal artery which supplies
the central grey matter of cord

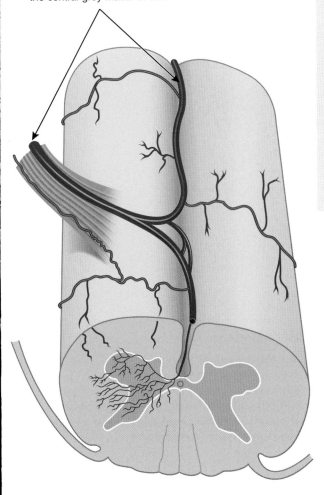

FIGURE 6.1 The blood supply of the lower cord and cauda equina

Diagram of the lower cord showing the 'great spinal artery' joining the anterior spinal artery to supply the lower cord. The upper parts of the spinal cord receive their blood supply from the vertebral arteries and their feeders. The cord terminates at L1–2 and its lower parts and the cauda equina receive their blood supply from the 'great spinal artery of Adamkievitz', a branch of a lower intercostal artery (often the 10th left intercostal artery).

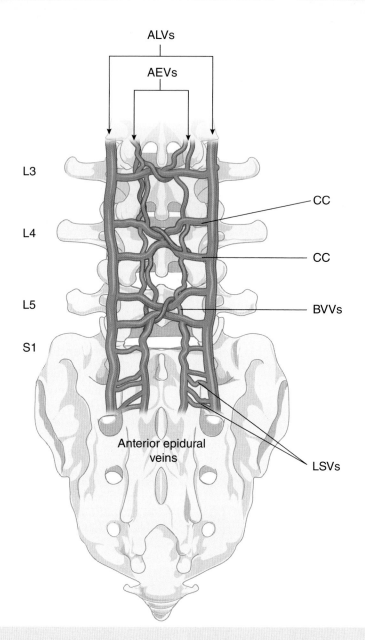

FIGURE 6.2 Veins of the spinal canal

The diagram of veins of the spinal canal is traced from venograms.

The paired, vertical, anterior epidural veins (AEVs) form a ladder pattern of valveless veins in the anterior epidural space of the spinal canal. Cross-connections (CC) of these valveless veins drain each vertebral body via the basi-vertebral veins (BVVs) from the centre of each vertebral body; they also connect with visceral and other structures outside the spinal canal by two veins passing through each intervertebral foramina to the ascending lumbar veins (ALVs). The lower end of the ALVs are renamed the lumbosacral veins (LSVs).

(C. McCormick, radiologist, personal communication)

CHAPTER 7

MUSCLES, LIGAMENTS, MOVEMENTS
(As Seen in Scans and Sections)

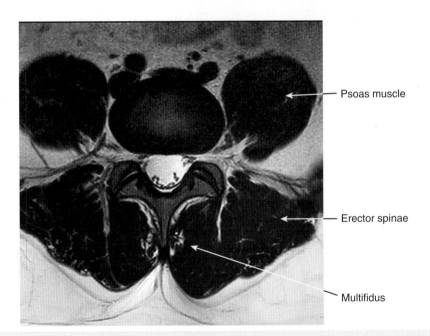

Psoas muscle

Erector spinae

Multifidus

FIGURE 7.1 A normal axial MRI section of lower lumbar joints and muscles

The extensor muscles (erector spinae and multifidus), as seen in axial views, fill the spaces between the spinous and transverse processes. The erector spinae lies lateral and its tendon lies superficial to and covers multifidus. Erector spinae arises from the back of the sacrum and from the posterior part of the iliac crest and its iliocostalis part ascends to attach to the lower six ribs near their angles. The medial part attaches to the tips of the lumbar spinous processes. The lumbar part of multifidus descends from the sides of spinous process passing obliquely down to attach to the mamillary process of facets two or three segments below. These lumbar extensor muscles are enclosed in a strong tendinous envelope.

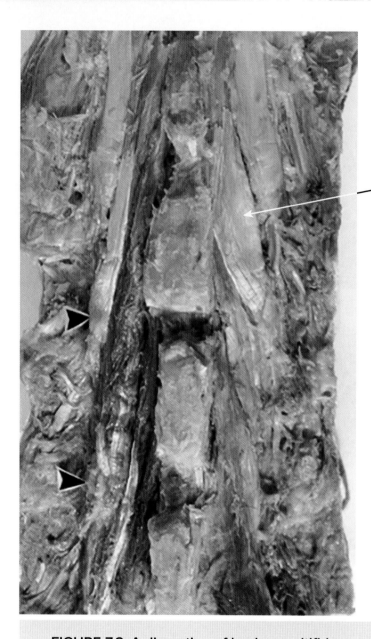

Part of an individual fascicle of multifidus

FIGURE 7.2 A dissection of lumbar multifidus

Dissection of individual fascicles of multifidus (see arrow-heads) shows their attachment to a spinous process above and into the mammillary process of a facet joint below.

Some fibres insert into the posterior capsule of the facet joint. This muscle is vulnerable to fatty change in chronic low-back-pain patients (Macintosh et al., 1986).

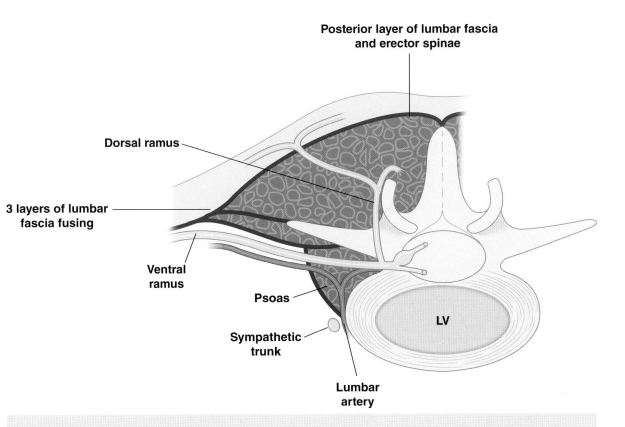

Posterior layer of lumbar fascia and erector spinae

Dorsal ramus

3 layers of lumbar fascia fusing

Ventral ramus

Psoas

Sympathetic trunk

Lumbar artery

LV

FIGURE 7.3 The lumbar fascia

The diagram shows erector spinae and multifidus enclosed in the posterior compartment of the lumbar fascia. This very strong collagenous envelope has separate anterior and posterior layers attached to the spinous and transverse processes respectively. These come together and fuse as one layer, lateral to the erector spinae. The abdominal muscles (internal oblique and transversus) are attached to this fascia, thus gaining attachment to the lumbar transverse and spinous processes. This allows them to act on individual lumbar vertebrae. Deep fibres of multifidus span one or two segments and can control individual motion segments. The external oblique and rectus abdominus have no vertebral attachments, but they brace the whole lumbar spine. Erector spinae fibres span many segments and cannot control individual motion segments. The anterior primary division of the segmental nerve passes between the innermost layer of the abdominal muscles (transversus abdominus) and the middle layer (internal oblique) to emerge through the rectus abdominus muscle.

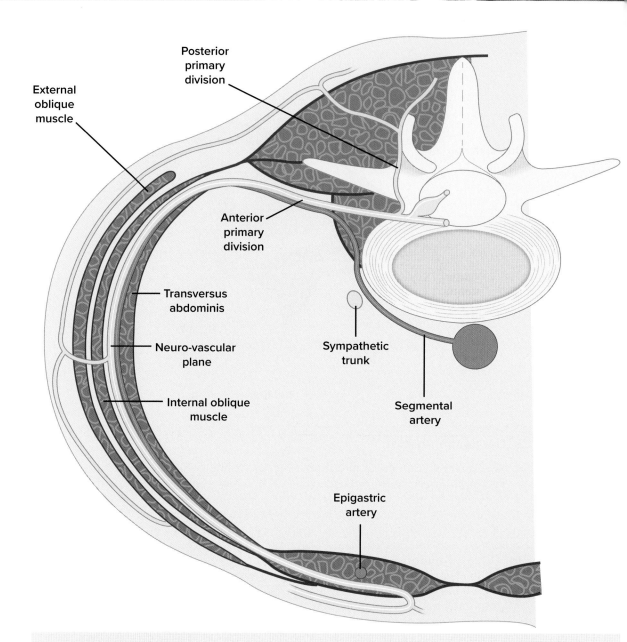

FIGURE 7.4 Abdominal muscles and the lumbar fascia

The transversus and internal oblique muscles are shown gaining attachment through the lumbar fascia to individual vertebrae.

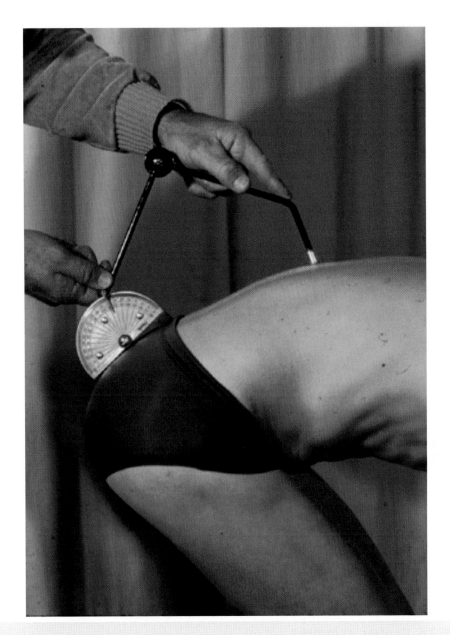

FIGURE 7.5 Ranges of lumbar spinal movement

Taylor and Twomey (1980) measured the lumbar ranges of movement in fresh cadaver specimens and in a living population. In cadavers, the average sagittal range was 52° in young adult females and 47° in young adult males. In living young adults, the sagittal range was 42° in both males and females. Axial rotation (one direction) was 15–18° in both adult males and females.

Axial rotation and anterior translation are resisted by facet joint orientation. The facets' restraint is less effective in a flexed spine. Both Twomey (1981) and Dvorak and colleagues (1991) have reviewed the topic of lumbar range of movement and give widely varying results (see Figure 7.6).

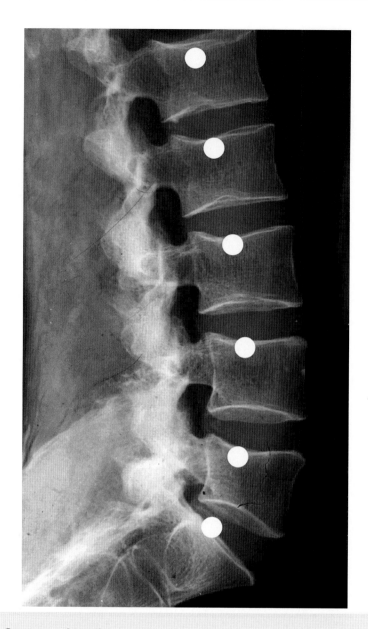

FIGURE 7.6 Centres of motion

The centres of motion for flexion and extension in the lumbar spine are located in the lower posterior disc or in the adjacent vertebral body, just below the disc (Aiyangar et al., 2017; Dvorak et al., 1991). A few millimetres of translation accompany rotation in the sagittal range (Kozanek et al., 2009). Dvorak and colleagues (1991) showed that the total sagittal range of forward and backward rotation of 76.9° was accompanied by 2–3 mm of translation at individual levels, except L5–S1. Dvorak also cited seven other studies which gave an average of 62.7° of sagittal ROM. L4–5 and L5–S1 are the most mobile individual segments at 15.5°. Lateral bending ROM was about 11° per segment from L1–2 to L4–5, with no lateral bending at L5–S1. This movement is not commonly used in life situations but is used in clinical assessment.

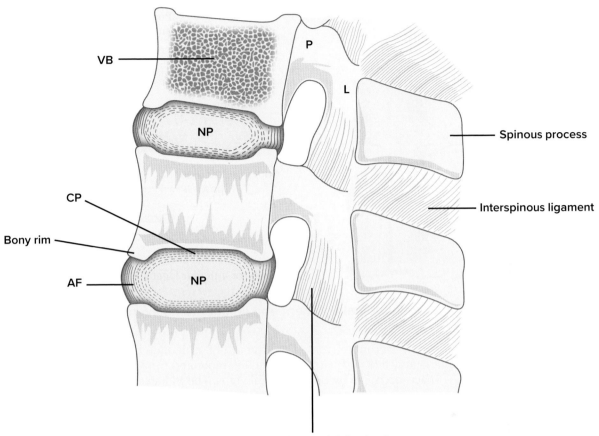

Labels on figure:
VB
P
L
NP
Spinous process
CP
Interspinous ligament
Bony rim
AF
NP
Ligamentum flavum joining laminae

FIGURE 7.7 Spinal ligaments

P = pedicle
VB = vertebral body
CP = cartilage plate
AF = annulus fibrosus
L = lamina

The ligamentum flavum (yellow ligament) and the interspinous ligament assist stability between the spinal segments.

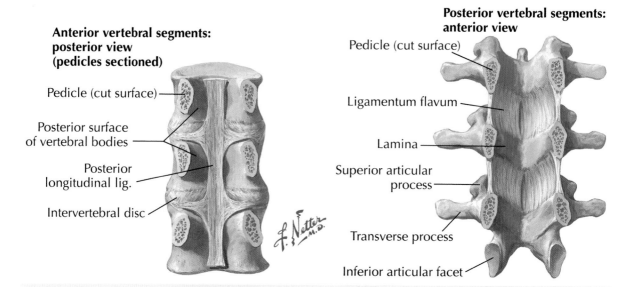

Anterior vertebral segments: posterior view (pedicles sectioned)

Pedicle (cut surface)

Posterior surface of vertebral bodies

Posterior longitudinal lig.

Intervertebral disc

Posterior vertebral segments: anterior view

Pedicle (cut surface)

Ligamentum flavum

Lamina

Superior articular process

Transverse process

Inferior articular facet

FIGURE 7.8 Posterior longitudinal ligament and ligamentum flavum

The pedicles are cut and the posterior longitudinal ligament (PLL) is viewed from behind; the ligamenta flava are viewed from in front. The lumbar PLL is dentate in shape, wide at the discs to which it is attached and narrow where it is separated from the back of the vertebral bodies by a space, occupied by basi-vertebral veins. The PLL extends from the sacrum to the foramen magnum.

The anterior longitudinal ligament (ALL) is a broad ribbon applied closely to the anterior surfaces of the discs and vertebrae. Its long fibres span several segments, extending from C1 to the sacrum (Cleland et al., 2015).

References

Aiyangar, A, Zheng, L, Anderst, W & Zhang, X 2017 Instantaneous centers of rotation for lumbar segmental extension in vivo. *Journal of Biomechanics*, 52, pp. 113–121. doi:10.1016/j.jbiomech.2016.12.021

Cleland, J, Koppenhaver, S and Su, J 2015 Netter's orthopaedic clinical examination: an evidence-based approach. Saunders, Philadelphia.

Dvorak, J, Panjabi, MM, Chang, DG et al. 1991 Functional radiographic diagnosis of the lumbar spine. Flexion-extension and lateral bending. *Spine*, 16(5), pp. 562–571. doi:10.1097/00007632-199105000-00014

Kozanek, M, Wang, S, Passias, PG et al. 2009 Range of motion and orientation of the lumbar facet joints in vivo. *Spine*, 34(19), pp. E689–696. doi:10.1097/BRS.0b013e3181ab4456

Macintosh, JE, Valencia, F, Bogduk, N & Munro, RR 1986 The morphology of the human lumbar multifidus. *Clinical Biomechanics*, 1(4), pp. 196–204. doi:10.1016/0268-0033(86)90146-4

Taylor, J & Twomey, L 1980 Sagittal and horizontal plane movement of the human lumbar vertebral column in cadavers and in the living. *Rheumatology*, 19(4), pp. 223–232. doi:10.1093/rheumatology/19.4.223

Twomey, LT 1981 Age changes in the human lumbar vertebral column. PhD Thesis.

CHAPTER 8

INNERVATION OF DISCS AND FACETS

LUMBAR DISCOGENIC PAIN

Knowledge of the innervation of lumbar discs is important to an understanding of discogenic low back pain. Pain provocation discography has been used to successfully identify a lumbar disc as a principal pain source (Bogduk, Aprill & Derby, 2013), but the adult lumbar intervertebral disc was long thought to be without appreciable innervation except in the outer lamellae of the annulus fibrosus (Bogduk, 1983; Cavanaugh, 1995).

Our dissection study found fine nerve filaments from the local spinal nerves; these entered the disc near the disc-vertebral body junction (epiphysis), and silver staining (Figure 8.3) showed nerve fibres penetrating six lamellae deep into the annulus.

In degenerate discs, fibres can be found deeper in the annulus and even in the nucleus (Freemont et al., 1997; Peng et al., 2005). Their pathways have also been studied using immunohistochemical techniques to demonstrate a dual pathway of afferent innervation involving the paravertebral sympathetic trunks non-segmentally and segmentally via the sinu-vertebral nerves and dorsal root ganglia (Edgar, 2007; Ohtori et al., 2015). The central vertebral endplate is a highly innervated structure and may be a potent source of discogenic pain (Fagan et al., 2003; Fields, Liebenberg & Lotz, 2014). Nerves supplying the endplate are said to originate from sinu-vertebral nerves and enter the vertebral bodies via the basi-vertebral foramen, branching with their nutrient arteries to reach the superior and inferior endplates (Bailey et al., 2011). Other developmental neurovascular channels may open up again conducting nerves to the endplates.

INNERVATION OF DISCS AND FACETS

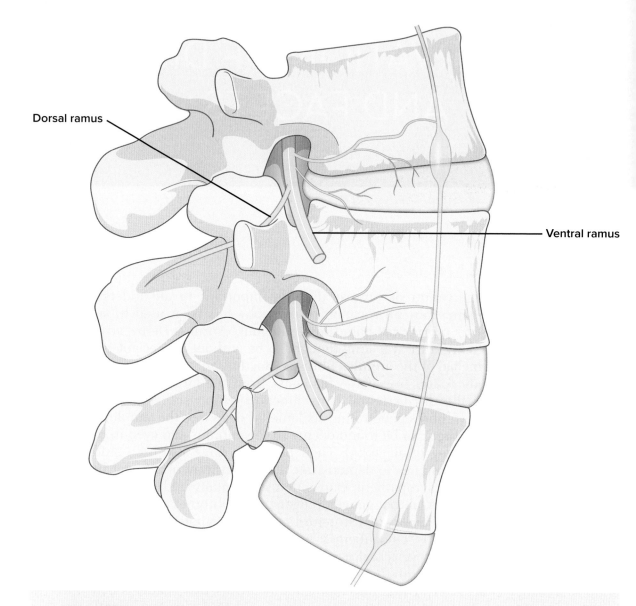

Dorsal ramus

Ventral ramus

FIGURE 8.1 Disc innervation

Each disc has direct branches from the ventral rami plus side branches from rami and communicates from the plexus of sinu-vertebral nerves.

VR = ventral ramus; DR = dorsal ramus

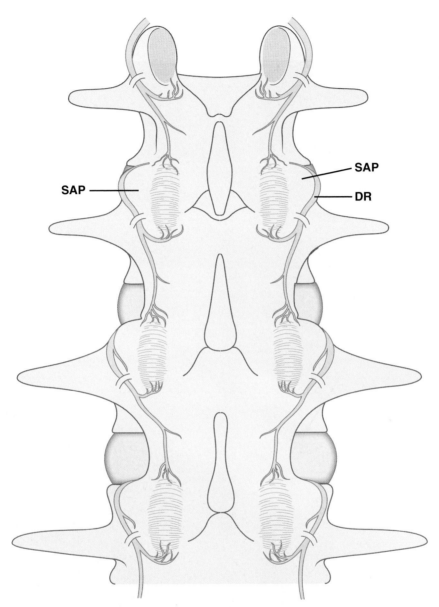

SAP

SAP

DR

**Branches of dorsal rami (DR) to
joint capsules and recesses**

FIGURE 8.2 Facet innervation

Each facet has dual innervation from medial branches of the dorsal rami.

VR = ventral ramus; DR = dorsal ramus; SAP = superior articular process.

This section of the outer layers of the annulus shows nerve fibres stained by silver. Nerve fibres were demonstrated up to six lamellae deep. Dr A.S. Wilson performed the silver staining of portions of fresh annulus, provided by J.Taylor. Similar images can be found in Bogduk, Tynan and Wilson (1981) and Ghannam and colleagues (2017).

INNERVATION OF LUMBAR FACET JOINTS

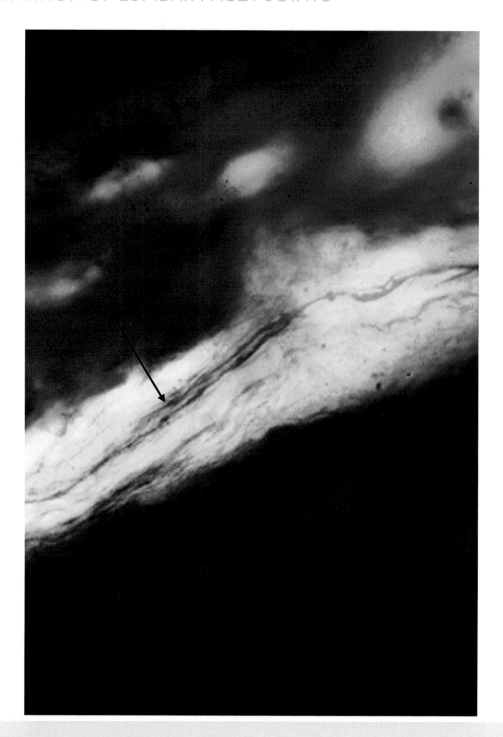

FIGURE 8.3 Nerve fibres in the annulus

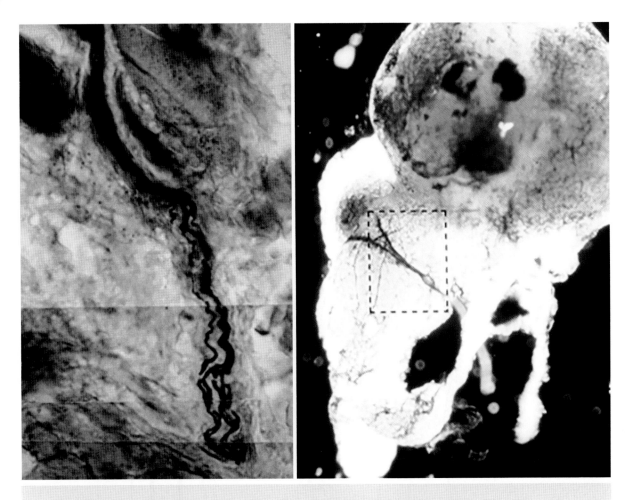

FIGURES 8.4 AND 8.5 Nerve fibres in the capsule and the base of facet synovial folds

Giles and Taylor (1987) used silver stains to demonstrate nerve fibres in the capsule and the base of facet synovial folds.

Figure 8.4 (left) shows nerve fibres in the fibrous capsule; Figure 8.5 (right) shows a nerve fibre in the base of a facet synovial fold (harvested with permission at surgery).

SEGMENTAL INNERVATION

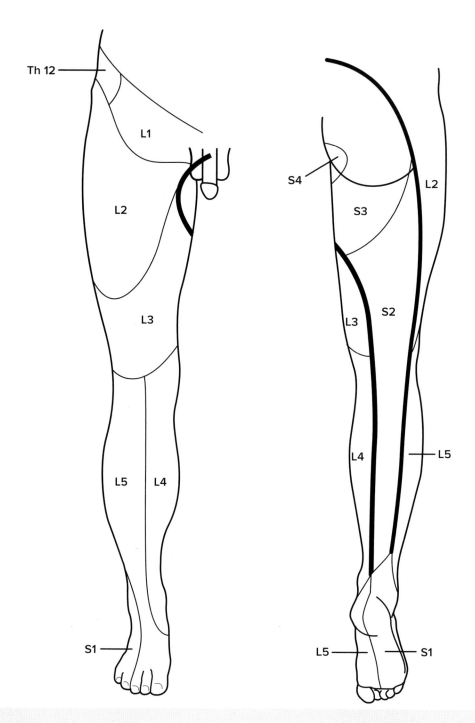

FIGURE 8.6 Dermatomes

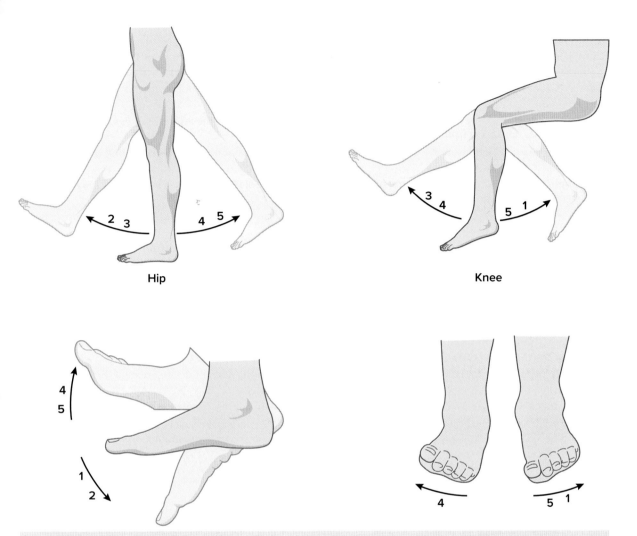

FIGURE 8.7 Myotomes

Sensory findings can vary between individuals, and segmental dermatome charts in the literature can have variation from author to author. However, the pattern is fairly standard and testing sensation in the dermatomes and power in the myotomes are important parts of clinical investigation.

Knowledge of segmental motor innervation can be most helpful in the clinical examination.

References

Bailey, JF, Liebenberg, E, Degmetich, S & Lotz, JC 2011 Innervation patterns of PGP 9.5-positive nerve fibers within the human lumbar vertebra. *Journal of Anatomy*, 218(3), pp. 263–270. doi:10.1111/j.1469-7580.2010.01332.x

Bogduk, N 1983 The innervation of the lumbar spine. *Spine*, 8(3), pp. 286–293. doi:10.1097/00007632-198304000-00009

Bogduk, N, Aprill, C & Derby, R 2013 Lumbar discogenic pain: state-of-the-art review. *Pain Medicine*, 14(6), pp. 813–836. doi:10.1111/pme.12082

Bogduk, N, Tynan, W & Wilson, AS 1981 The nerve supply to the human lumbar intervertebral discs. *Journal of Anatomy*, 132(1), pp. 39–56.

Cavanaugh, JM 1995 Neural mechanisms of lumbar pain. *Spine*, 20(16), pp. 1804–1809. doi:10.1097/00007632-199508150-00011

Edgar, MA 2007 The nerve supply of the lumbar intervertebral disc. *Journal of Bone & Joint Surgery, British*, 89(9), pp. 1135–1139. doi:10.1302/0301-620X.89B9.18939

Fagan, A, Moore, R, Vernon Roberts, B et al. 2003 ISSLS prize winner: The innervation of the intervertebral disc: a quantitative analysis. *Spine*, 28(23), pp. 2570–2576. doi:10.1097/01.BRS.0000096942.29660.B1

Fields, AJ, Liebenberg, EC & Lotz, JC 2014 Innervation of pathologies in the lumbar vertebral end plate and intervertebral disc. *Spine*, 14(3), pp. 513–521. doi:10.1016/j.spinee.2013.06.075

Freemont, AJ, Peacock, TE, Goupille, P et al. 1997 Nerve ingrowth into diseased intervertebral disc in chronic back pain. *Lancet*, 350(9072), pp. 178–181. doi:10.1016/s0140-6736(97)02135-1

Ghannam, M, Jumah, F, Mansour, S et al. 2017 Surgical anatomy, radiological features, and molecular biology of the lumbar intervertebral discs. *Clinical Anatomy*, 30(2), pp. 251–266. doi:10.1002/ca.22822

Giles, LG & Taylor, JR 1987 Human zygapophyseal joint capsule and synovial fold innervation. *British Journal of Rheumatology*, 26(2), pp. 93–98. doi:10.1093/rheumatology/26.2.93

Ohtori, S, Inoue, G, Miyagi, M & Takahashi, K 2015 Pathomechanisms of discogenic low back pain in humans and animal models. *Spine*, 15(6), pp. 1347–1355. doi:10.1016/j.spinee.2013.07.490

Peng, B, Wu, W, Hou, S et al. 2005 The pathogenesis of discogenic low back pain. *Journal of Bone & Joint Surgery, British*, 87(1), pp. 62–67.

Further reading

Aoki, Y, Ohtori, S, Takahashi, K et al. 2004 Innervation of the lumbar intervertebral disc by nerve growth factor-dependent neurons related to inflammatory pain. *Spine*, 29(10), pp. 1077–1081. doi:10.1097/00007632-200405150-00005

Coppes, MH, Marani, E, Thomeer, RT et al. 1990 Innervation of annulus fibrosis in low back pain. *Lancet*, 336(8708), pp. 189–190. doi:10.1016/0140-6736(90)91723-n

Groen, GJ, Baljet, B & Drukker, J 1990 Nerves and nerve plexuses of the human vertebral column. *American Journal of Anatomy*, 188(3), pp. 282–296. doi:10.1002/aja.1001880307

Ohtori, S, Takahashi, K, Yamagata, M et al. 2001 Neurones in the dorsal root ganglia of T13, L1 and L2 innervate the dorsal portion of lower lumbar discs in rats. A study using dil, an anterograde neurotracer. *Journal of Bone & Joint Surgery, British*, 83(8), pp. 1191–1194. doi:10.1302/0301-620x.83b8.11012

CHAPTER 9

ANATOMICAL VARIANTS CAUSING 'WEAK POINTS'

Three structural 'weak points' are illustrated in Chapter 9.

1. There is a developmental 'weak point' at the centre of the cartilage endplates in young thoraco-lumbar vertebral columns. Schmorl's nodes often occur here in adolescents while the nucleus pulposus is still 'fluid' enough to herniate into the adjacent vertebral body.
2. There is an associated, relative weakness along the linear junction of the cartilaginous intervertebral disc with the bony vertebral body (Taylor, 2017). This weakness in the mid and lower thoracic spine and the upper lumbar spine may allow aberrant herniation of the nucleus pulposus into the growth plates of adolescents; these atypical Schmorl's nodes would deform the vertebral bodies.
3. The lower lumbar pars interarticularis is vulnerable to high loading, due to erect posture with a marked lower lumbar lordosis. Stress fractures commonly occur here in adolescents or young adults especially in athletes performing elite sports like fast bowling or gymnastics.

SCHMORL'S NODES AND SCHEUERMANN'S DEFORMITIES

Schmorl's nodes are among the most common variants seen in the mid and lower thoracic spine and the upper lumbar spine. Schmorl's nodes are due to herniation of soft nucleus pulposus material into a vertebral body, through a weak point in the centre of the cartilage endplate where the notochord originally passed through the foetal spine. At this point, the cartilage endplate is only half the average cartilage endplate thickness: The Schmorl's nodes occur in adolescents when the nucleus pulposus is still fluid enough to herniate.

Development of Schmorl's nodes

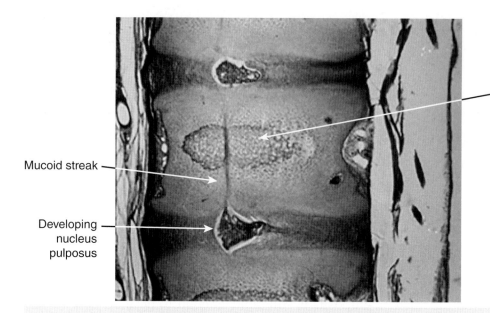

Mucoid streak

Developing nucleus pulposus

The primary centre of ossification is appearing in the cartilage model of a vertebral body. The track of the notochord is marked by the mucoid streak passing through it.

FIGURE 9.1 The course of the notochord in a 75 mm fetus

The nucleus pulposus is formed in a human fetus when the rapid growth of the vertebral body 'squeezes out' the notochordal tissue into the developing disc. The notochordal tissue aggregates in the disc to form the nucleus pulposus, leaving only a 'mucoid streak' where the notochord originally passed through the vertebral bodies.

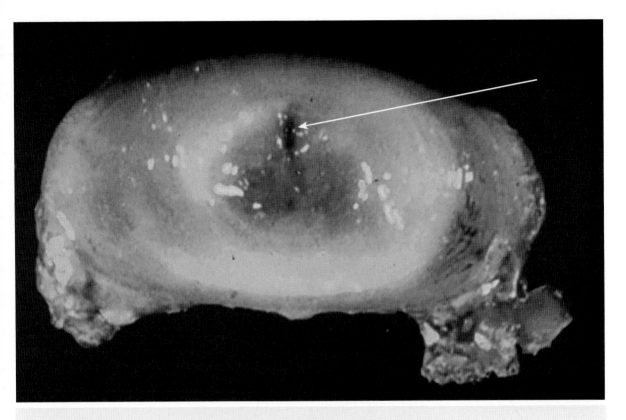

FIGURE 9.2 A transverse section of a still-born infant disc

The transverse section shows a dimple-shaped 'defect' (see arrow) in the midline of the cartilage endplate. It appears as a dark depression where the cartilage endplate thickness is reduced to about half of the cartilage endplate thickness elsewhere.

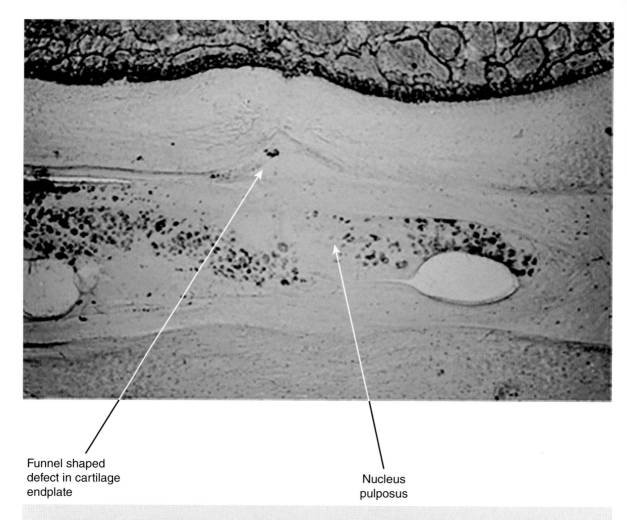

Funnel shaped
defect in cartilage
endplate

Nucleus
pulposus

FIGURE 9.3 In a 100-micron mid-sagittal section of an infant disc the dimple appears as a triangular defect in the cartilage endplate

The 'dimple' in the cartilage endplate, where the notochord passed through the vertebral column in the fetus, can still be found in mid-sagittal sections of fetuses and children; it persists into adolescence. This defect or weak point in the cartilage endplate is the site of a Schmorl's node, with part of the nucleus pulposus herniating through the CP into the vertebral body spongiosa (Taylor, 1974).

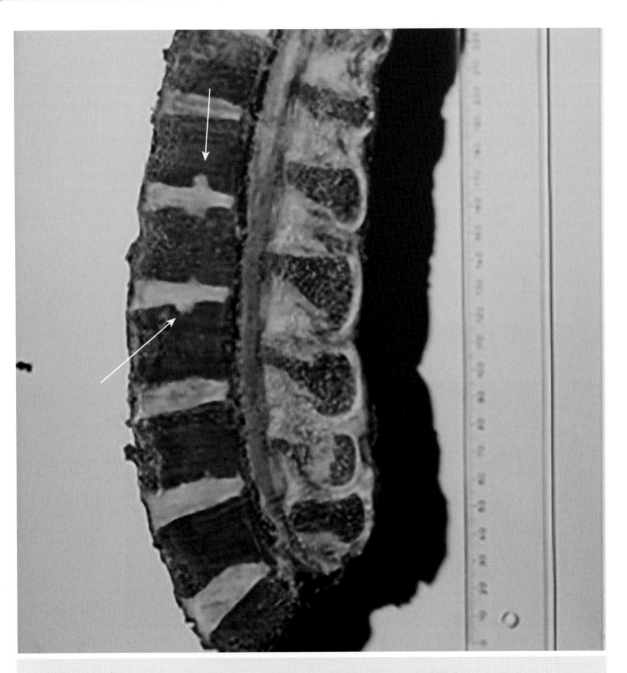

FIGURE 9.4 Schmorl's nodes in a young adult midline section

Schmorl's nodes aligned with each other along the original line of the notochord, in a midline section of the thoraco-lumbar spine (Twomey, 1981).

The multiple Schmorl's nodes are aligned with each other, along the line of the original notochord.

Schmorl examined and sectioned thousands of autopsy spines and found Schmorl's nodes in 38% of adult columns in the mid and lower thoracic, and upper lumbar vertebrae. They were more common in males (40%) than in females (34%). He suggested that the herniations occurred through the central developmental weak points due to the loading stresses of everyday life and work in apprentice adolescents (Schmorl & Junghans, 1971).

Taylor and Twomey (1986a) examined 80 thoracolumbar x-rays from normal subjects and 110 autopsy lumbar spines for Schmorl's nodes. There were no Schmorl's nodes in children but 15% of adolescents showed Schmorl's nodes on x-rays and 25% of autopsy specimens showed Schmorl's nodes; 21% of adult x-rays and 30% of adult autopsy specimens showed Schmorl's nodes. Schmorl's nodes only 'show up' on x-rays if there is sufficient bony reaction around the nucleus pulposus hernia.

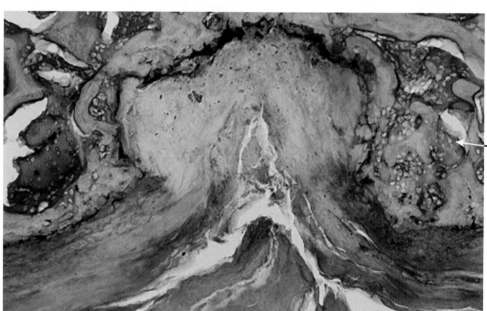

Increased vascular tissue

FIGURE 9.5 A typical Schmorl's node in a stained 100-micron, mid-sagittal section from an adolescent male aged 16 years

The deep purple staining at the junction of the node with the vertebral spongiosa is due to the reactive calcification and new bone formation. There is also increased vascularity (greeny-yellow) around the Schmorl's node vertebral body interface (Taylor & Twomey, 1986b).

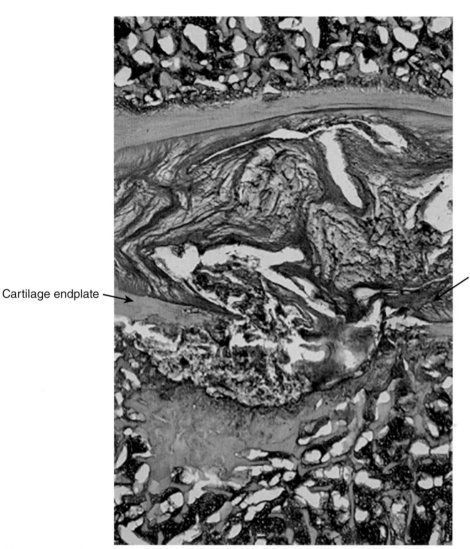

Cartilage endplate

The herniation (red) is tracking through a fracture in the cartilage endplate.

FIGURE 9.6 An atypical Schmorl's node from a 16-year-old male subject, showing herniated nucleus pulposus material (red) spreading horizontally at the bone-cartilage interface

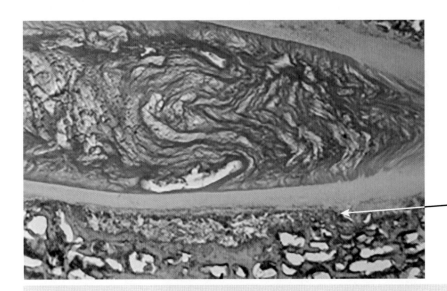

The pink-stained herniated nucleus pulposus material is tracking between the cartilage endplate and the bony endplate, where it would destroy the growth plate.

FIGURE 9.7 Spread of herniated nucleus pulposus material along the bone-cartilage interface

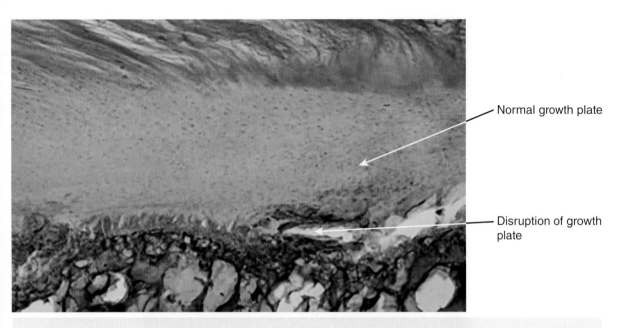

Normal growth plate

Disruption of growth plate

FIGURE 9.8 The growth plate in a higher-power magnification

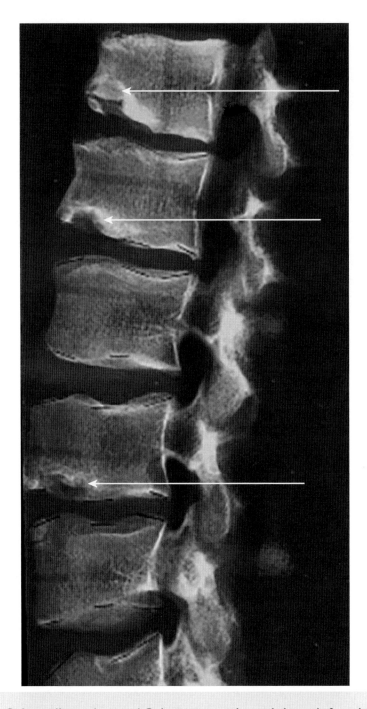

FIGURE 9.9 Schmorl's nodes and Scheuermann's endplate deformities: An x-ray of the thoraco-lumbar spine in a young adult shows the endplate deformities of Scheuermann's disease

ABERRANT SCHMORL'S NODES AND ENDPLATE DEFORMITIES

Schmorl noted an association between the presence of multiple Schmorl's nodes and the likelihood of Scheuermann's deformities in the same spines, but he was unable to find the mechanism of deformity. The Schmorl's nodes themselves are not clinically significant but it is possible in a few individuals that herniations may deviate along the bone-cartilage interface, damaging the growth plate (Schmorl & Junghans, 1971). McFadden and Taylor (1989) found increased vascularity in the regions immediately around Schmorl's nodes. They suggested that the increased vascularity around Schmorl's nodes may cause further endplate changes. It should be noted that the bone-cartilage interface has been shown to be a 'weak point' in studies of injuries to the cervical spine (Taylor, 2017).

The case above shows deviation of a Schmorl's node along the relatively weak bone-cartilage junction at the endplate. This can only occur in young people where the nucleus pulposis remains relatively fluid. If similar herniations occur at multiple levels in the thoracic spine they may cause Scheuermann's kyphotic deformity.

Lumbar vertebral bodies grow like long bones at the growth plate between the shaft (diaphysis) and the epiphysis. The vertebral epiphysis of humans is cartilaginous, unlike quadrupeds (for example, sheep), which have a bony plate epiphysis. The 'weak point' in adolescents, described above, includes the growth plate for growth in vertebral height. Herniation of the soft nucleus pulposus of a child would disrupt growth in height producing a deformed vertebral body and possibly a deformed spine.

There is a linear weakness at the cartilage joint with the bony vertebral body at the epiphyseal diaphyseal junction. If nucleus pulposus tissue herniates into the growth plate in immature subjects it will stop or disrupt growth causing an irregular endplate. This would constitute a mechanism for an irregular endplate in the lumbar spine and Scheuermann's deformity in the thoracic spine.

PARS INTERARTICULARIS FRACTURES AND SPONDYLOLYSIS

The 'weak point' described here is in the pars interarticularis of lower lumbar vertebrae which may fail due to overloading in hyper-lordotic exercise; for example, in athletes such as fast bowlers (Hardcastle et al., 1992) or female gymnasts (Jackson, Wiltse & Cirincoine, 1976). This stress fracture is called 'spondylolysis'. It is not an age change as it occurs in adolescents and young adults, and it is found in 5% of lumbar spines as a variant related to the adoption of erect posture and participation in sporting and other activities that overload the lower lumbar pars interarticularis.

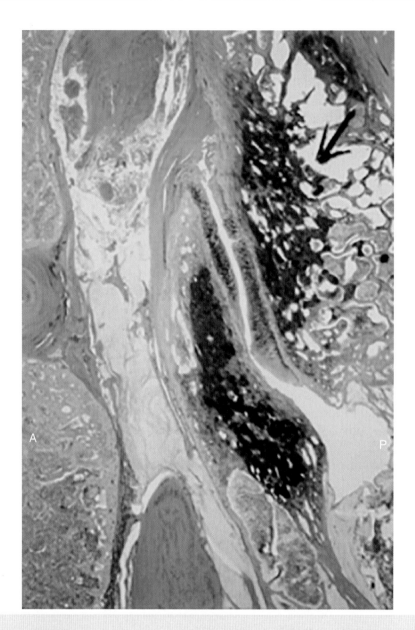

FIGURE 9.10 A 100-micron stained sagittal section of lower lumbar facets from a 17-year-old adolescent

The dense purple staining pattern, due to increased bone density, illustrates the pathway of forces through the facet joint and to the pars interarticularis. The dense staining pattern shows the direction of transmission of loading through the facets. The articular cartilages in this line show increased chondrocyte activity and darker staining in the pathway of load transmission.

A = anterior

P = posterior

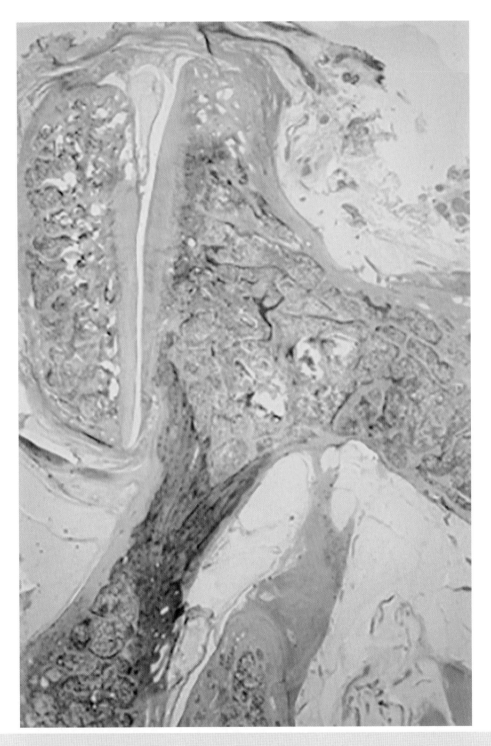

FIGURE 9.11 A sagittal section of an adolescent lower lumbar facet joint with the pars interarticularis below. The dense staining of bone in the pars indicates the reaction to loading

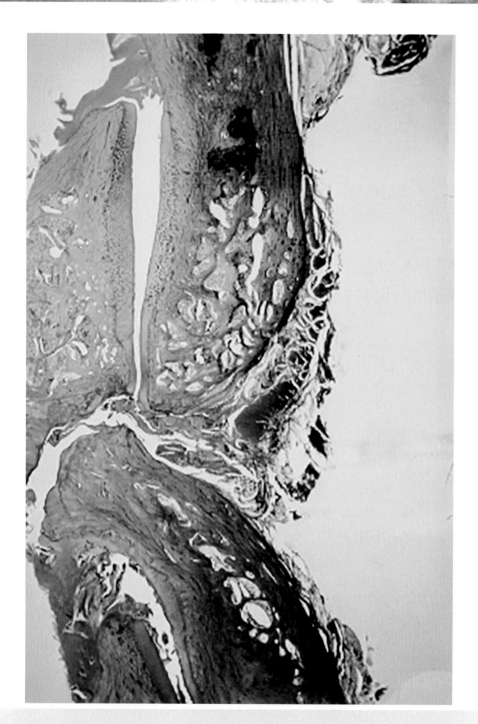

FIGURE 9.12 A lower lumbar spondylolysis in sagittal section from a 17-year-old boy

The lower lumbar pars interarticularis from a 17-year-old adolescent male shows an undisplaced stress fracture with fibrous change (green) covering both ends of the fractured bone. This could act as an extra, accessory joint. In addition to the spondylolysis, there is forward bending of the pars, due to remodelling of the pars.

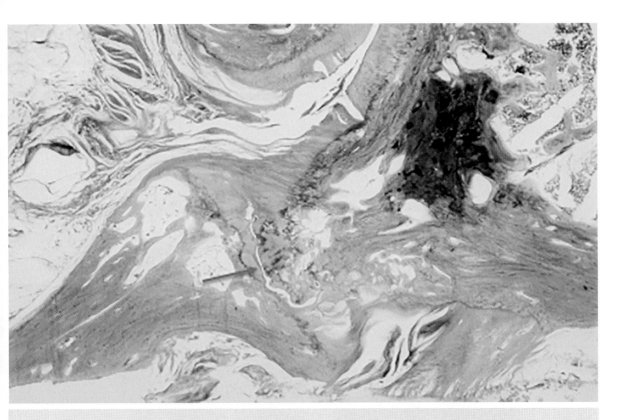

FIGURE 9.13 Transverse section of a spondylolysis in a young adult male

Arrow show a pars interarticularis fracture with abnormal healing.

This spondylolysis resembles an osteo-arthritic joint with fibrous union around the expanded irregular fracture surfaces.

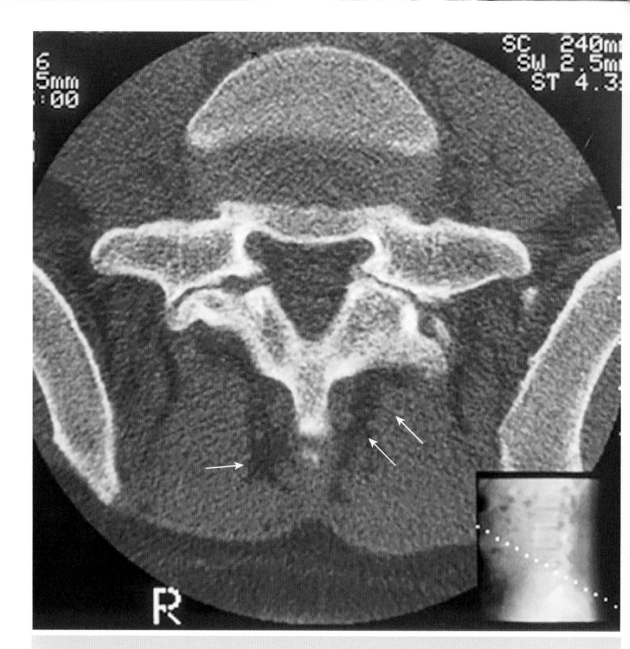

FIGURE 9.14 A reverse gantry CT of bilateral spondylolysis in a young adult patient with low back pain

The reverse gantry angle CT shows bilateral undisplaced spondylolysis. The expanded end surfaces at the fracture resemble a false joint. There is medial fatty change in the multifidus muscles (arrow indicates the dark area of fatty infiltration).

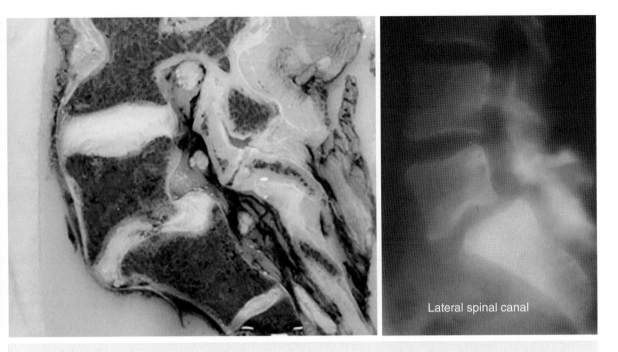

Lateral spinal canal

FIGURES 9.15 AND 9.16 Examples of spondylolytic olisthesis in sagittal section and lateral view

Normal facet orientation protects the disc from injury but when this protection is lost due to bilateral spondylolysis, the disc is subject to sheer forces likely to cause degeneration with forward slip (olisthesis) of the upper vertebra on the lower vertebra. There is forward bending of the pars at the fracture line in both cases (Ohmori et al., 1995; Saraste, 1993).

References

Hardcastle, P, Annear, P, Foster, DH et al. 1992 Spinal abnormalities in young fast bowlers. *Journal of Bone & Joint Surgery, British*, 74(3), pp. 421–425. doi:10.1302/0301-620X.74B3.1587894

Jackson, DW, Wiltse, LL & Cirincoine, RJ 1976 Spondylolysis in the female gymnast. *Clinical Orthopaedics and Related Research*, (117), pp. 68–73.

McFadden, KD & Taylor, JR 1989 End-plate lesions of the lumbar spine. *Spine*, 14(8), pp. 867–869. doi:10.1097/00007632-198908000-00017

Ohmori, K, Ishida, Y, Takatsu, T et al. 1995 Vertebral slip in lumbar spondylolysis and spondylolisthesis. Long-term follow-up of 22 adult patients. *Journal of Bone & Joint Surgery, British*, 77(5), pp. 771–773.

Saraste, H 1993 Spondylolysis and spondylolisthesis. *Acta Orthopaedica Scandinavica* Supplement 251, pp. 84–86. doi:10.3109/17453679309160129

Schmorl, G & Junghans, H 1971 *The human spine in health and disease*. Grune & Stratton, New York.

Taylor, J 1974 Growth and development of human intervertebral discs. PhD thesis.

Taylor, J 2017 *The cervical spine*. Elsevier, Australia.

Taylor, JR & Twomey, LT 1986a Age changes in lumbar zygapophyseal joints. Observations on structure and function. *Spine*, 11(7), pp. 739–745. doi:10.1097/00007632-198609000-00014

Taylor, JR & Twomey, LT 1986b The role of the notochord and blood vessels in development of the vertebral column. In Grieve, G (ed.), *Grieve's modern manual therapy: The vertebral column*. Churchill Livingstone, London.

Twomey, LT 1981 Age changes in the human lumber vertebral column. PhD thesis.

CHAPTER 10

AGE CHANGES

AGE CHANGES IN VERTEBRAL BODIES: OSTEOPOROSIS

In old age there is shortening in the thoracic and in the lumbar spine, not so much from reduced disc thickness but rather due to osteoporosis in the vertebral bodies. In the vertebral bodies we noted changed internal structure with initial loss of transverse trabeculae. The consequent loss of support and reduced rigidity of the vertical trabeculae allows them to bend under load, to the point of fracture so that the vertebral endplates collapse with increased endplate concavity and loss of stature (Twomey, Taylor & Furniss, 1983).

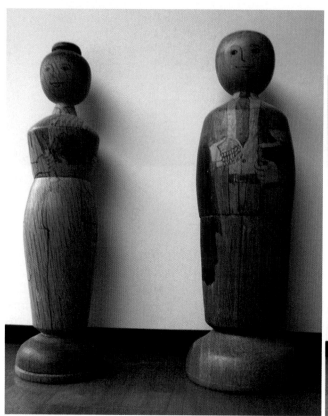
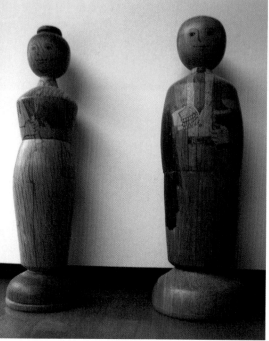

25 years   80 years

FIGURE 10.1 Loss of stature with ageing

Twomey, Taylor and Furniss (1983) measured decreased bone density in lumbar vertebral bodies with ageing. They found that horizontal trabeculae were lost first, causing loss of stiffness in the vertical trabeculae that support the endplates, leading to endplate collapse into increased concavity. Loss of stature with ageing is due, in part, to this increased endplate concavity and to increased kyphosis in the thoracic spine.

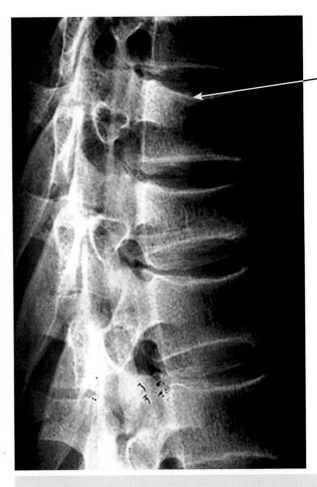

There is collapse of thoracic vertebral endplates with marked increase in their concavity. The increased penetration of x-rays makes the porotic central vertebral bodies appear darker, while the dense endplates, by contrast, appear white. Similar, less advanced changes are seen in the lumbar vertebrae. Loss of height in the thoracic vertebral bodies causes increased kyphosis, contributing to the loss of stature.

Osteoporosis is common. The lifetime risk of osteoporotic fracture in the USA was reported as 40% in white women and 13% in white men (Lenchik & Sartoris, 1997), with vertebral fractures being the most common osteoporotic fracture (Chen et al., 2009). In a European study, the incidence of vertebral fracture was approximately 5 (males) to 10 (females) per 1000 person years in 60- to 64-year-olds, rising to 12 (males) to 30 (females) per 1000 person years in the 74- to 79-year-old age group (European Prospective Osteoporosis Study et al., 2002; L.T. Twomey & Taylor, 1987).
Two-thirds of Australians aged over 50 years are said to have osteoporosis or osteopenia (Watts, Abimanyi-Ochom & Sanders, 2013).

FIGURE 10.2 Osteoporotic collapse of vertebral bodies in the thoraco-lumbar spine

In Twomey's 1981 study of vertebral body changes with age, in a general population study, there was evidence of vertebral body osteopenia with increased concavity of the vertebral endplates with increased disc height centrally and decreased disc height peripherally.

Regular exercise and adequate calcium intake reduces the risk of severe osteoporosis.

AGE CHANGES IN INTERVERTEBRAL DISCS

Given the primary changes of increased vertebral endplate concavity, there is a reciprocal increase in disc convexity at the vertebral endplates. Comparing young and old discs, we have measured a loss of proteoglycans (PG) and water with ageing (Scott et al., 1994) which results in a greater tendency to creep on loading in older discs with delayed recovery (hysteresis). This makes the lumbar spine of older people less able to withstand high loading in manual work. It is also common to observe in lumbar discs of older subjects, disc bulging at the posterior margin and an increase in circumferential and radial disc fissuring (Osti et al., 1992).

Lumbar disc degeneration (LDD)

Gross studies

Twomey's extensive 'general population' study (1981) found minimal age-related degenerative changes in upper lumbar discs but there was loss of disc height and fissuring in 33% of the L4–5 and L5–S1 discs. In his midline sectioning study of 204 cadaver spines of all ages, Twomey found that one-third of the L4–5 and L5–S1 discs from subjects over 60 years of age showed severe degeneration. However, Kramer (1981) found disc space narrowing in only 17% of 244 adult lumbar spines and he found no significant increased narrowing in old age.

Microscopic studies

Farfan (1973) found lumber disc degeneration in 70% of 182 cadaver spines, with most L4–5 and L5–S1 discs showing annular fissures. Vernon-Roberts and Pirie (1977) also found splits and clefts in the annulus of many elderly spines, while Scott and colleagues (1994) observed a decrease in the proteoglycan content of lumbar discs with increase in age.

The nerve roots exit the spinal canal through the upper part of the intervertebral foramen, at some distance above the disc and facet joint. Age-related fissuring of the inner annulus and nucleus pulposus may not be painful as the nucleus and inner annulus are not normally innervated. However, it has been shown that inner parts of the disc may become innervated by ingrowth of nerves and vessels when there is a damaged endplate.

When the nucleus and inner annulus remain enclosed by outer annulus and vertebral endplates, the disc still behaves hydrostatically under load (Nachemson & Elfstrom, 1970). Internal disc disruption with acute tearing of the outer, innervated third of the annulus is likely to be painful, especially if there is accompanying inflammatory change (Gunzburg et al., 1992).

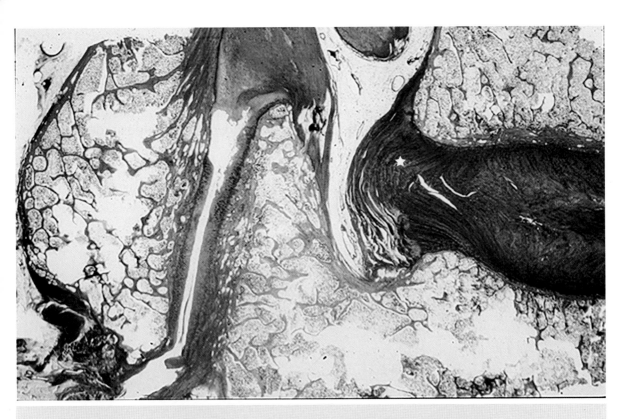

FIGURE 10.3 Sagittal section of a lumbar disc showing a disc bulge

A posterior disc 'bulge' or protrusion is common and usually asymptomatic.

Disc fissuring

Disc fissuring was classified by Osti and colleagues (1992) as peripheral, circumferential or radiating. In their study of 135 post-mortem lumbar discs, peripheral tears were most frequent in the anterior annulus, circumferential tears were found equally in the anterior and posterior annulus and radiating tears were found mostly in the posterior annulus. Radiating tears were closely related to the presence of severe nucleus pulposus degeneration.

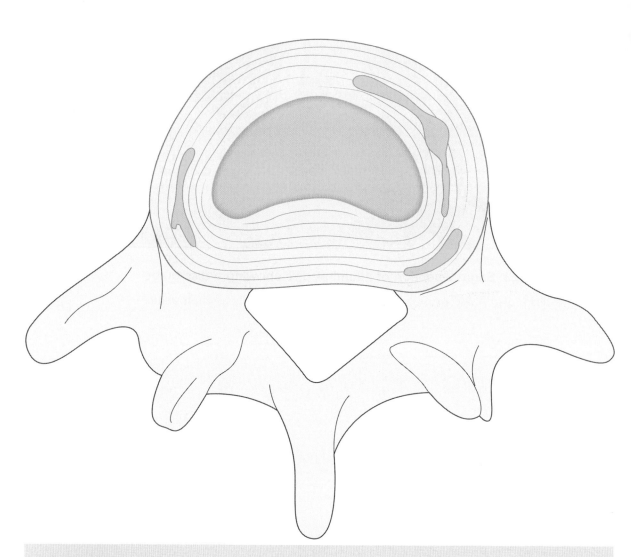

FIGURE 10.4 Diagram of an axial discogram showing circumferential fissuring of a lumbar annulus

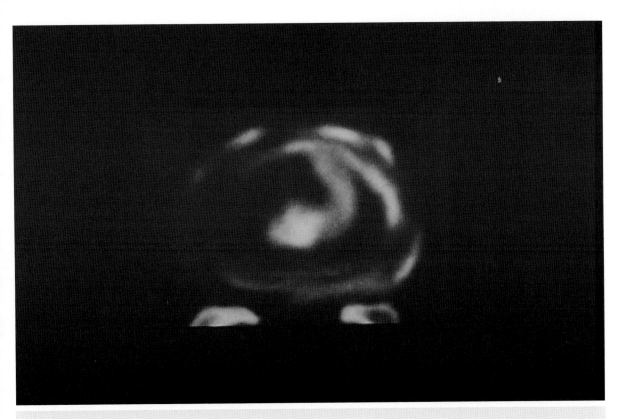

FIGURE 10.5 An axial discogram showing spread of contrast from the nucleus through inner and outer annular fissures

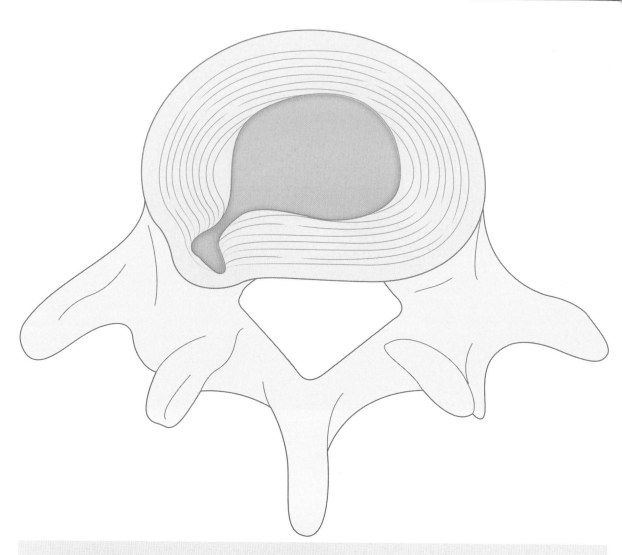

FIGURE 10.6 A diagram of an axial discogram showing a radial tear extending into the outer innervated third of the annulus

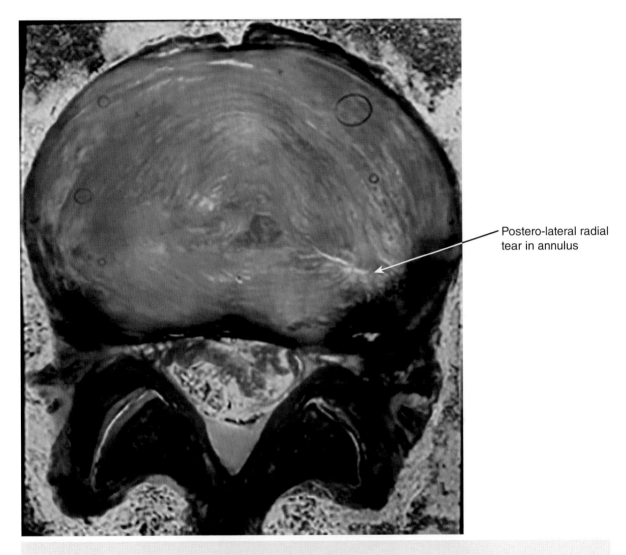

Postero-lateral radial tear in annulus

FIGURE 10.7 Transverse section of a lumbar disc with a radial fissure

Radial fissures have been associated with low back pain (Osti et al., 1992).

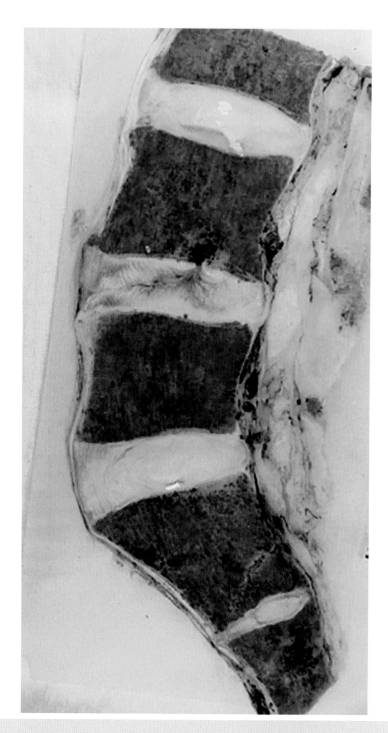

FIGURE 10.8 Sagittal section of a lumbar spine from a 69-year-old man

In this otherwise healthy lumbar spine, damage to the endplate/disc junction allows ingrowth of vessels and nerves into the central parts of the L4–5 disc (Freemont et al., 1997, 2002).

AGE CHANGES IN LUMBAR FACET JOINTS

Studies of sections of post-mortem lumbar facet joints show the appearance of chondromalacia, predominantly affecting the anterior third of the superior articular facet. This part of the facet is oriented close to the coronal plane and subject to higher compressive loading in bending and lifting activities. This loading also causes thickening of the subchondral bone late in the anterior third of lumbar facet joints. With increasing age, we often found bony hypertrophy of the facets with marginal osteophytes and sclerosis in the anterior coronal parts of the superior articular processes. In old age, cartilage loss was common as a feature of osteoarthritis.

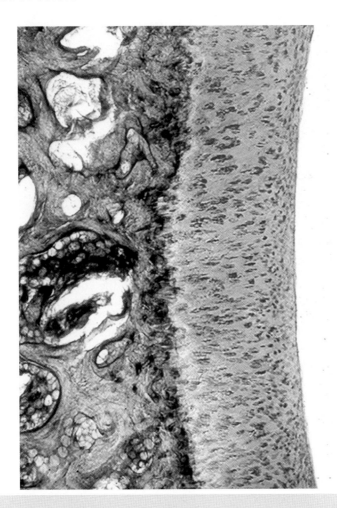

FIGURE 10.9 Stained, 100-micron transverse section of normal facet articular cartilage from a young adult

This shows healthy chondrocytes, a beautifully smooth articular surface, and a thin calcified layer joining it to the vascular subchondral bone plate. The long axis of the oval chondrocytes lies perpendicular to the joint surface, corresponding to the predominant collagen fibre orientation.

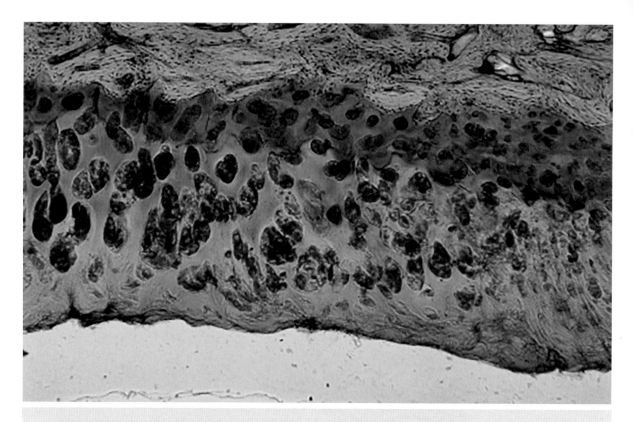

FIGURE 10.10 Stained transverse section of lumbar facet articular cartilage from a middle-aged adult male

This articular cartilage does not appear thinner than in the young articular cartilage, but its deep calcified layer is thicker (purple), joining it to the more dense, less vascular subchondral bone. The thicker, deep, calcified layer makes the articular cartilage even more dependent on nutrition from the synovial fluid that bathes its surface. Regular movement is essential for circulation of synovial fluid through the cartilage (Taylor & Twomey, 1986; Tobias, Ziv & Maroudas, 1992).

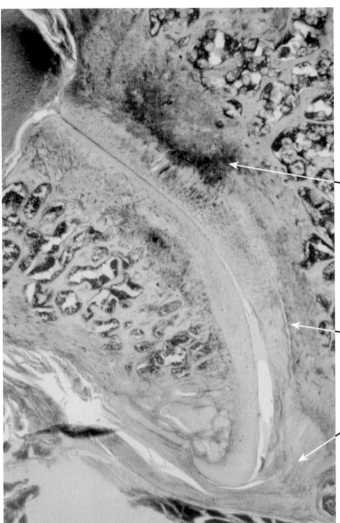

This shows the beginnings of sclerotic change due to compressive loading in the anterior part of the subchondral bone plate of the superior articular facet. This area shows increased staining of chondrocytes and a few splits in the articular cartilage.

Split appearing along the bone cartilage junction

Posterior capsule

FIGURE 10.11 Transverse section of the posterior part of the lumbar facet from a 36-year-old adult male

Note the long fibres of the posterior capsule in direct continuity with the posterior margin of the articular cartilage of the superior facet. Traction effects appear to be tearing the posterior articular cartilage away from the bone.

Despite the greater compressive loading of the anterior part of the joint leading to chondromalacia, in middle life (55+ years) it is often the posterior part of the superior facet that loses its articular cartilage. The direct attachment of the posterior fibrous capsule into the posterior margin of the articular cartilage (lower arrow) means that in movement it would exert traction on the articular cartilage, with shearing along the articular cartilage bone interface (upper arrows).

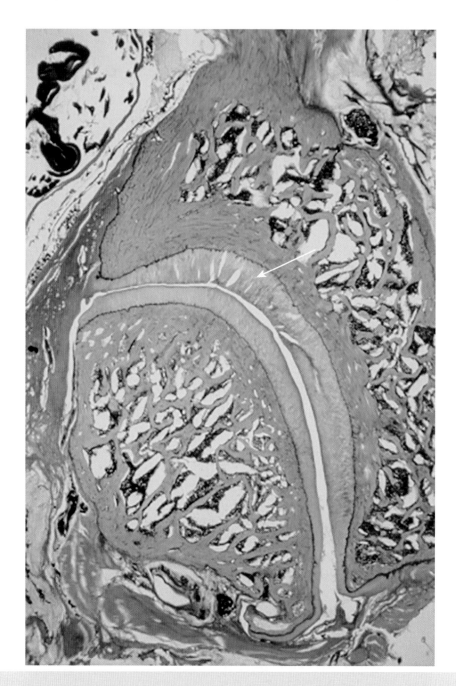

FIGURE 10.12 Stained 100-micron transverse section of a facet joint from a different 36-year-old adult showing chondromalacia

This shows chondromalacia in the anterior third of the superior articular facet (see arrow) with multiple splits in the articular cartilage. The splits are perpendicular to the articular cartilage bone junction corresponding to the internal collagen framework of the articular cartilage. This is a frequent finding in middle age; its frequency, nature and position show that it is not an artefact.

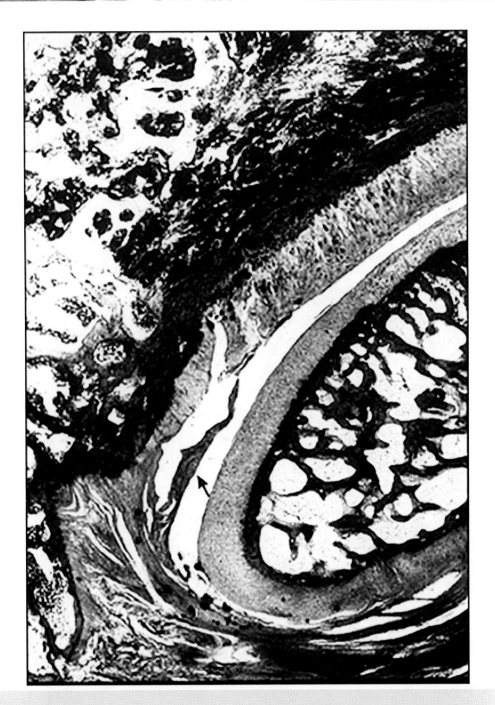

FIGURE 10.13 A loose flap of articular cartilage in a transverse section of a lumbar facet joint

There is extensive formation of new cartilage around the posterior margin of the inferior facet, which appears to be 'rubbing on' the thickened posterior fibrous capsule. Part of the articular cartilage has become detached from the superior articular facet forming a loose flap, which is capable of being displaced within the joint, perhaps 'locking' the joint.

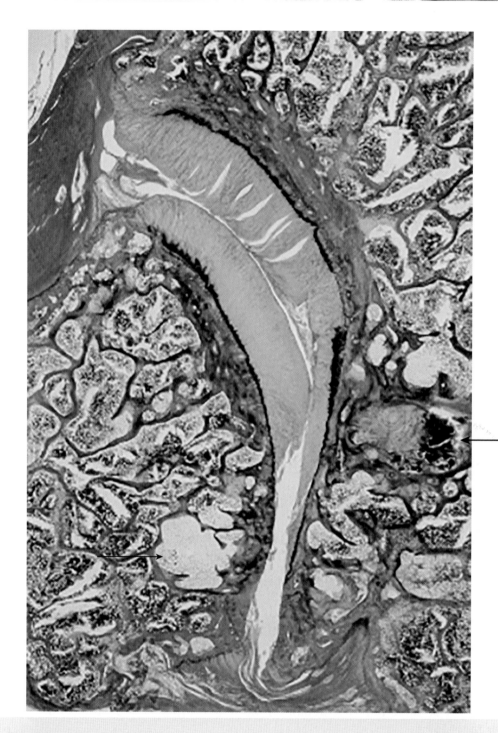

FIGURE 10.14 Transverse section of a lumbar facet joint (61-year-old male), showing osteoarthrosis with subchondral bone cysts (arrows)

There is extensive loss of articular cartilage from the posterior articular surfaces, with two subchondral bone cysts, typical of osteoarthrosis in other synovial joints.

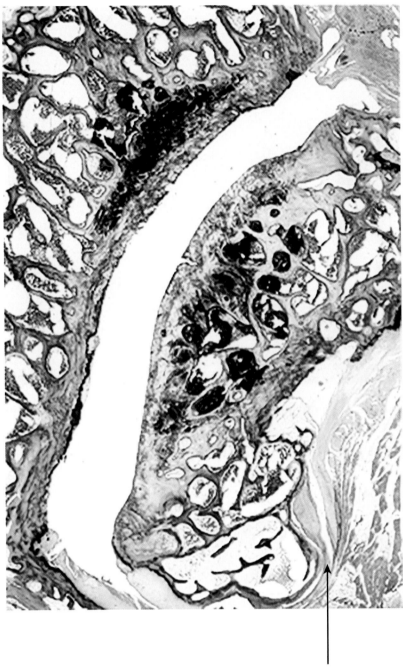

An osteophyte, growing
from the posterior articular
margin of the inferior
articular process

FIGURE 10.15 Complete loss of articular cartilage with articular sclerosis in a 100-micron stained transverse section of a lumbar facet joint from a 74-year-old

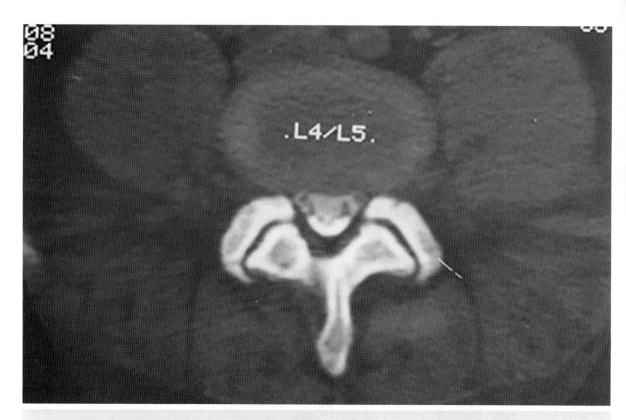

FIGURE 10.16 An axial CT scan at L4–5 showing facet hypertrophy with marginal osteophytes

The osteophytes enlarge the superior facets. The darker appearance deep to multifidus, behind the lamina, suggests some replacement of muscle by fat.

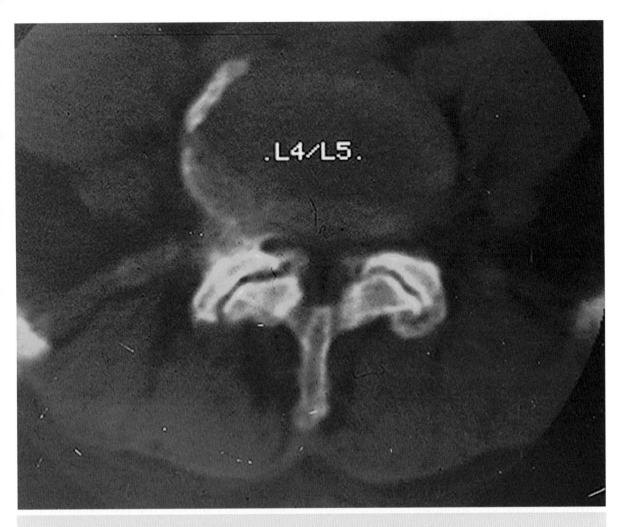

FIGURE 10.17 An axial CT image of L4–5 from an elderly patient

There are gross changes with facet enlargement and deformity in the facets due to osteoarthritis.

There is extensive fatty change in posterior muscles.

Facet size in osteoarthrosis

We measured superior facet size from anterior to posterior margin in 200 axial CTs (Taylor & Taylor, unpublished study). These showed an average 25% enlargement between 25 years and 65 years. This was accompanied by partial loss of joint space. Gross facet enlargement appeared to be a cause of spinal stenosis.

Age-related changes in range of movement

These changes apply to the whole motion segment:
- With increasing age there is increased **stiffness** and associated reduction in **ranges of movement**. Further, there is increased **creep and delayed hysteresis**.
- Twomey's cadaver studies (1981) showed a significant decline of average sagittal ROM from:
  - 47° (young men) to 34° (men over 60)
  - 52° (young women) to 36° (women over 60).
- In an extensive study in living subjects in the Busselton survey comparing young people with elderly subjects there was reduction in average sagittal ROM from: 42° to 30° in men and from 42° to 28° in women (Figure 10.18). This resembled average reductions with increase in age in other studies (Dvorak et al., 1991; Scott et al., 1994; Taylor & Twomey, 1980).

With increase in age there is:
- reduced range of movement
- increased creep
- delayed hysteresis (recovery from creep).

(Creep is the progressive deformation of a structure under prolonged loading: loss of proteoglycans causes increased creep with prolonged loading and delayed recovery. Hysteresis is the recovery from distortion after the load has been removed.)

Twomey and Taylor (1982) demonstrated an increase in creep and a delay in hysteresis with advancing age in adult unfixed cadaver spines. This reflects the reduction in disc proteoglycans with ageing (Scott et al., 1994). The proteoglycans have the function of holding water in the tissue. Loss of proteoglycans makes it easier for loading to squeeze out water and harder for the tissue to rehydrate after removal of load.

Axial creep

Normal subjects of all ages show reduction in stature of about 1.5 cm during the course of the day's normal activities due to squeezing of water out of the discs, a change which is reversed when recumbent at night (De Puky, 1935; Stone, 1983).

While testing normal sagittal plane movements in cadavers, Twomey measured the restraining effect of the posterior ligaments and facets. The most effective restraints of flexion at normal end range were the facets (Twomey & Taylor, 1983).

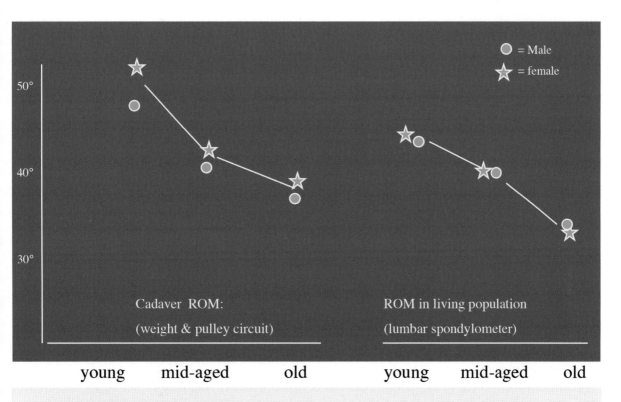

FIGURE 10.18 Different sagittal range of movement in three age groups

Taylor & Twomey, 1980

SUMMARY OF AGE CHANGES OBSERVED

- Reduced length of the lumbar spine with ageing is mainly due to osteoporosis or osteopenia with bowing of the lumbar endplates. Most upper lumbar discs preserve a normal 'naked-eye' appearance in old age but one-third of L4–5 and L5–S1 discs show severe degenerative changes in subjects over 60 years of age.
- There is progressive loss of sagittal range of movement with increase in age. Loss of disc proteoglycans with ageing results in increased creep with reduced rate of recovery on removing the load. We found reduced lumbar lordosis and increased thoracic kyphosis in old age, associated with loss of vertebral body height. Both bone loss and postural change contribute to reduced stature.
- Discogenic pain may be due to radial fissuring of lower lumbar intervertebral discs in the innervated outer annulus; pain may also follow ingrowth of vessels and nerves into the central disc through vertebral endplate lesions.
- Spinal stenosis may result from gross facet hypertrophy and gross disc degeneration or from segmental instability with likelihood of sciatica and lower limb muscle atrophy.
- Chronic low back pain is often accompanied by low back muscle wasting, especially of multifidus, much of which could be prevented by suitable exercise programs so long as there is not already nerve damage due to chronic pressure on spinal nerves.

(Crock, 1986; Kong et al., 2009; Lundon & Bolton, 2001; Nagaosa et al., 1998; O'Sullivan et al., 1997; Osti & Fraser, 1992; Schwarzer et al., 1994; Taylor, Twomey & Levander, 2000; Taylor et al., 1992; Twomey & Taylor, 1982)

References

Chen, P, Krege, JH, Adachi, JD et al. 2009 Vertebral fracture status and the World Health Organization risk factors for predicting osteoporotic fracture risk. *Journal of Bone and Mineral Research*, 24(3), pp. 495–502. doi:10.1359/jbmr.081103

Crock, HV 1986 Internal disc disruption. A challenge to disc prolapse fifty years on. *Spine*, 11(6), pp. 650–653.

De Puky, P 1935 The physiological oscillation of the length of the body. *Acta Orthopaedica Scandinavica*, 6(1–4), pp. 338–347. doi:10.3109/17453673508991358

Dvorak, J, Panjabi, MM, Chang, DG et al. 1991 Functional radiographic diagnosis of the lumbar spine. Flexion-extension and lateral bending. *Spine*, 16(5), pp. 562–571. doi:10.1097/00007632-199105000-00014

European Prospective Osteoporosis Study (EPOS) Group, Felsenberg, D, Silman, AJ et al. 2002 Incidence of vertebral fracture in Europe: results from the European Prospective Osteoporosis Study (EPOS). *Journal of Bone and Mineral Research*, 17(4), pp. 716–724. doi:10.1359/jbmr.2002.17.4.716

Farfan, H 1973 *Mechanical disorders of the low back*. Lea and Febiger, Philadelphia.

Freemont, AJ, Peacock, TE, Goupille, P et al. 1997 Nerve ingrowth into diseased intervertebral disc in chronic back pain. *Lancet*, 350(9072), pp. 178–181. doi:10.1016/s0140-6736(97)02135-1

Freemont, AJ, Watkins, A, Le Maitre, C et al. 2002 Nerve growth factor expression and innervation of the painful intervertebral disc. *Journal of Pathology*, 197(3), 286–292. doi:10.1002/path.1108

Gunzburg, R, Parkinson, R, Moore, R et al. 1992 A cadaveric study comparing discography, magnetic resonance imaging, histology, and mechanical behavior of the human lumbar disc. *Spine*, 17(4), pp. 417–426. doi:10.1097/00007632-199204000-00007

Kong, MH, Morishita, Y, He, W et al. 2009 Lumbar segmental mobility according to the grade of the disc, the facet joint, the muscle, and the ligament pathology by using kinetic magnetic resonance imaging. *Spine*, 34(23), pp. 2537–2544. doi:10.1097/BRS.0b013e3181b353ea

Kramer, J 1981 *Intervertebral disc lesions: causes, diagnosis, treatment and prophylaxis.* Georg Thieme, Stuttgart.

Lenchik, L & Sartoris, DJ 1997 Current concepts in osteoporosis. *American Journal of Roentgenology*, 168(4), pp. 905–911. doi:10.2214/ajr.168.4.9124138

Lundon, K & Bolton, K 2001 Structure and function of the lumbar intervertebral disk in health, aging, and pathologic conditions. *Journal of Orthopaedic & Sports Physical Therapy*, 31(6), pp. 291–303; discussion pp. 304–296. doi:10.2519/jospt.2001.31.6.291

Nachemson, A & Elfstrom, G 1970 Intravital dynamic pressure measurements in lumbar discs. A study of common movements, maneuvers and exercises. *Scandinavian Journal of Rehabilitation Medicine Supplement*, 1, pp. 1–40.

Nagaosa, Y, Kikuchi, S, Hasue, M & Sato, S 1998 Pathoanatomic mechanisms of degenerative spondylolisthesis. A radiographic study. *Spine*, 23(13), pp. 1447–1451. doi:10.1097/00007632-199807010-00004

O'Sullivan, PB, Phyty, GD, Twomey, LT & Allison, GT 1997 Evaluation of specific stabilizing exercise in the treatment of chronic low back pain with radiologic diagnosis of spondylolysis or spondylolisthesis. *Spine*, 22(24), pp. 2959–2967. doi:10.1097/00007632-199712150-00020

Osti, OL & Fraser, RD 1992 MRI and discography of annular tears and intervertebral disc degeneration. A prospective clinical comparison. *Journal of Bone & Joint Surgery, British*, 74(3), pp. 431–435. doi:10.1302/0301-620X.74B3.1587896

Osti, OL, Vernon-Roberts, B, Moore, R & Fraser, RD 1992 Annular tears and disc degeneration in the lumbar spine. A post-mortem study of 135 discs. *Journal of Bone & Joint Surgery, British*, 74(5), pp. 678–682. doi:10.1302/0301-620X.74B5.1388173

Schwarzer, AC, Aprill, CN, Derby, R et al. 1994 The relative contributions of the disc and zygapophyseal joint in chronic low back pain. *Spine*, 19(7), pp. 801–806. doi:10.1097/00007632-199404000-00013

Scott, JE, Bosworth, TR, Cribb, AM & Taylor, JR 1994 The chemical morphology of age-related changes in human intervertebral disc glycosaminoglycans from cervical, thoracic and lumbar nucleus pulposus and annulus fibrosus. *Journal of Anatomy*, 184(1), pp. 73–82.

Stone 1983 Honours thesis. University of Western Australia, Australia.

Taylor, JR & Twomey, LT 1980 Sagittal and horizontal plane movement of the human lumbar vertebral column in cadavers and in the living. *Rheumatology and Rehabilitation*, 19(4), pp. 223–232. doi:10.1093/rheumatology/19.4.223

Taylor, JR & Twomey, LT 1986 Age changes in lumbar zygapophyseal joints. Observations on structure and function. *Spine*, 11(7), pp. 739–745. doi:10.1097/00007632-198609000-00014

Taylor, J, Twomey, L & Levander, B 2000 Contrasts between cervical and lumbar motion segments. *Critical Reviews in Physical and Rehabilitation Medicine*, 12(4), pp. 345–371. doi:10.1615/critrevphysrehabilmed.v12.i4.40

Taylor, JR, Scott, JE, Cribb, AM & Bosworth, TR 1992 Human intervertebral disc acid glycosaminoglycans. *Journal of Anatomy*, 180(1), pp. 137–141.

Tobias, D, Ziv, I & Maroudas, A 1992 Human facet cartilage: swelling and some physico-chemical characteristics as a function of age. Part 1: Swelling of human facet joint cartilage. *Spine*, 17(6), pp. 694–700.

Twomey, LT 1981 Age changes in the human lumber vertebral column. PhD thesis, University of Western Australia, Australia.

Twomey, LT & Taylor, JR 1982 Flexion creep deformation and hysteresis in the lumbar vertebral column. *Spine*, 7(2), pp. 116–122. doi:10.1097/00007632-198203000-00005

Twomey, LT & Taylor, JR 1983 Sagittal movements of the human lumbar vertebral column: a quantitative study of the role of the posterior vertebral elements. *Archives of Physical Medicine and Rehabilitation*, 64(7), pp. 322–325.

Twomey, LT & Taylor, JR 1987 Age changes in lumbar vertebrae and intervertebral discs. *Clinical Orthopaedics and Related Research*, (224), pp. 97–104.

Twomey, LT, Taylor, JR & Furniss, B 1983 Age changes in the bone density and structure of the lumbar vertebral column. *Journal of Anatomy*, 136(1), pp. 15–25.

Vernon-Roberts, B & Pirie, CJ 1977 Degenerative changes in the intervertebral discs of the lumbar spine and their sequelae. *Rheumatology and Rehabilitation*, 16(1), pp. 13–21. doi:10.1093/rheumatology/16.1.13

Watts, JJ, Abimanyi-Ochom, J & Sanders, KM 2013 *Osteoporosis costing all Australians. A new burden of disease analysis, 2012–2022*. Retrieved from https://healthybonesaustralia.org.au/wp-content/uploads/2020/11/Burden-of-Disease-Analysis-2012-2022.pdf

CHAPTER 11

SEVERE DEGENERATION AND INSTABILITY

SEGMENTAL STABILITY

The discs are by far the strongest structures in the motion segment, but they need intact facets and healthy muscles to protect them from injury. The lumbar facets are oriented to protect the disc from shearing forces in translation and torsion, with support in different postures and movement by the segmental muscles. When the disc is severely injured or degenerate, so that it no longer forms a tight, stable, well-aligned joint between adjacent vertebral bodies, normal movements are lost and the innervated parts of the annulus become painful on movement (Farfan & Gracovetsky, 1984; O'Sullivan et al., 1997).

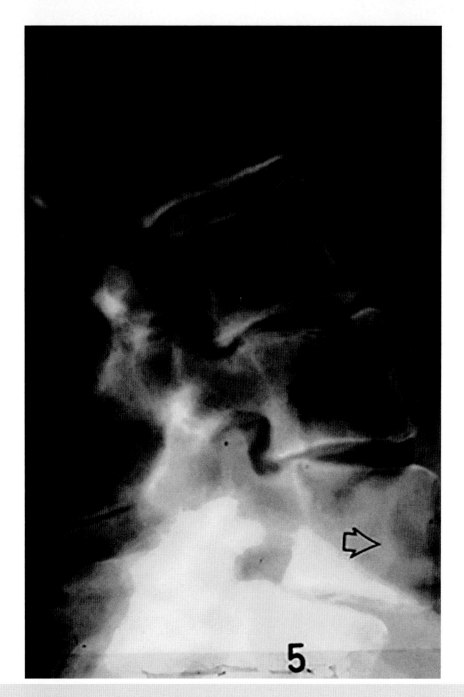

FIGURE 11.1 Multi-level instability

The x-ray (from Dr C. McCormick at Royal Perth Hospital) shows multi-level instability with loss of disc spaces and abnormal position of vertebral bodies. There is gross instability with anterolisthesis of L5 and retrolisthesis of L4 and L3. The intervertebral joints no longer maintain correct alignment, the facet joint articular surfaces no longer fit correctly, and the facet tips intrude into the upper intervertebral foramina.

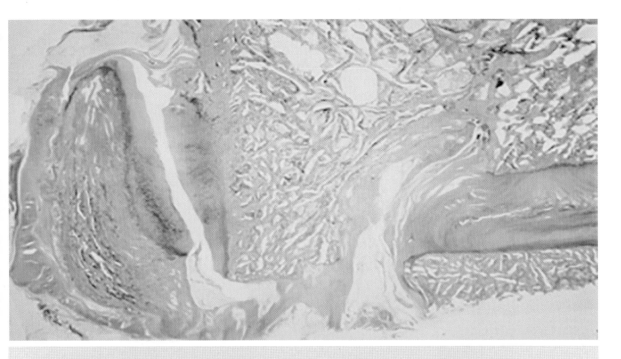

FIGURE 11.2 Segmental instability in a stained 100-micron sagittal section from a 57-year-old man

A lumbar facet joint and the posterior parts of the vertebral bodies and disc are shown. The disc is degenerate and severely deformed so that there is retrolisthesis of the upper vertebra on the lower vertebra, so that the facets are subluxed with the inferior articular process (IAP) of the upper vertebra subluxed backwards and downwards. The IAP does not articulate closely with the superior articular process of the vertebra below (Farfan & Gracovetsky, 1984; Lehmann & Brand, 1983; O'Sullivan et al., 1997; Taylor, Taylor & McCormick, 1992).

Instability of one or more lumbar motion segments is associated with low back pain (LBP) in 20–30% of LBP patients (Kotilainen et al., 1997; Lehmann & Brand, 1983; Schwarzer et al., 1994; Taylor, Twomey & Levander, 2000; Tokuhashi, Matsuzaki & Sano, 1993).

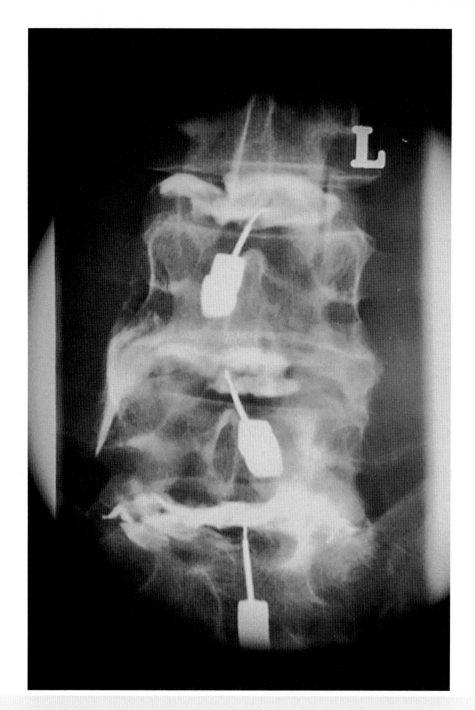

FIGURE 11.3 Internal disc disruption demonstrated by discography

Centrally injected contrast has spread through disc fissures in L3–4, L4–5 and L5–S1, leaking out on the surface of the vertebral column.

The discograms (from Dr P. Finch) show severe multi-level degeneration with fissuring.

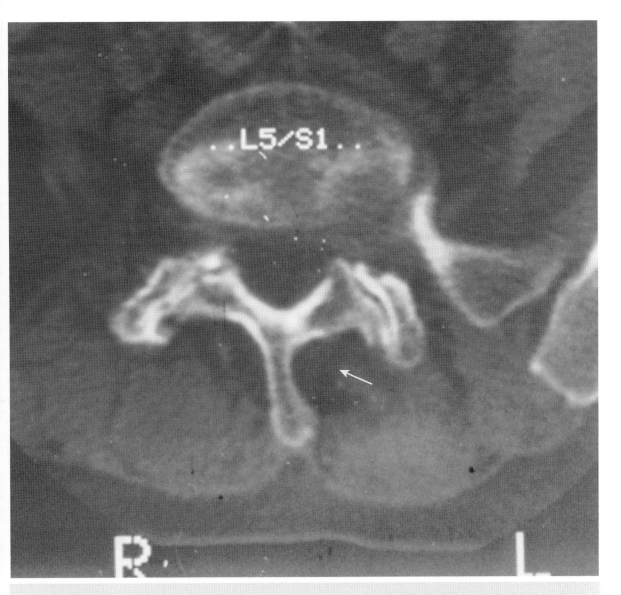

FIGURE 11.4 Degenerative spondylolisthesis in a 72-year-old woman

The enlarged facets are arthritic and the disc is degenerate, allowing the sagittally oriented inferior articular process to slide forwards on the superior articular process. There is extensive bilateral fatty change in deep parts of multifidus (arrowhead) (Wang & Yang, 2009).

Spondylolytic olisthesis

In Figures 9.11 to 9.13 (on pages 85–87) the staining patterns in these adolescent and young adult specimens suggested transmission of loading through the facets and the pars interarticularis. The articular cartilage chondrocytes also showed increased staining in the pathway of load transmission. The pars showed increased bone density. In 5% of cases, a stress fracture (spondylolysis) occurs.

In patients with bilateral spondylolysis, the facets no longer protect the disc from shear forces in forward translation so that the disc degenerates and the motion segment becomes unstable with forward slip of the upper vertebra (Beutler et al., 2003; Hardcastle et al., 1992; O'Sullivan et al., 1997; Ohmori et al., 1995; Teplick et al., 1986).

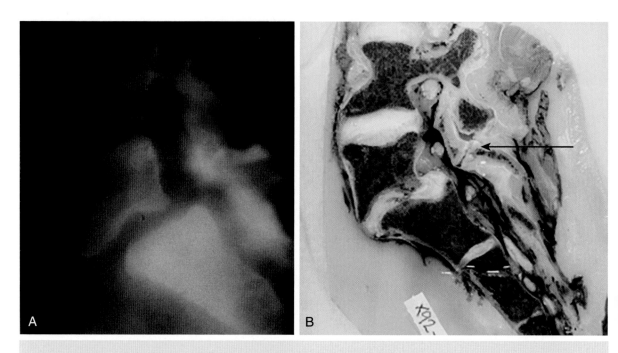

A   B

FIGURES 11.5A AND 11.5B Spondylolysis with forward slip or olisthesis of L5 in two young adults

The L5 pars is bent forwards and the degenerate disc allows olisthesis of L5 on S1.

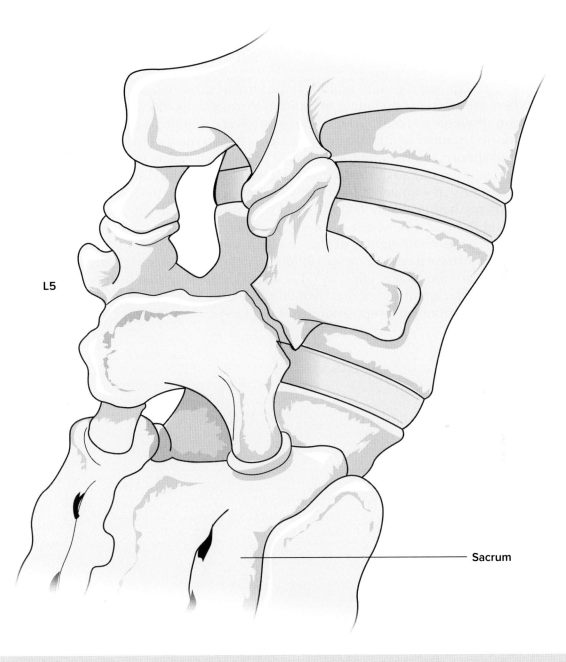

FIGURE 11.5C Spondylolysis can be demonstrated in an oblique x-ray of an affected spine

The diagram of the oblique-view x-ray shows the fracture line in the pars; this appearance resembles a 'scotty dog' wearing a collar.

INSTABILITY IN OLDER SUBJECTS

Lumbar rotational strain

Farfan (1973) recognised the vulnerability of the lumbar spine to torsion forces, especially in flexion where the facets are no longer in position to protect the disc from torsion. In manual examination of whole unfixed lumbar spines, we were unable to detect unstable motion segments during manual sagittal plane movements but on manual twisting in axial rotation we identified abnormal movement with loss of the normal elastic recoil in a small number of spines, most often in L4–5, due to gross degeneration of the disc in older subjects and due to severe injury in younger subjects (Taylor, Taylor & McCormick, 1992). The abnormal motion segments had probably been injured in a rotational strain. Placing each suspect spine in a simple apparatus, which allowed CT scanning of the spine in left and right axial rotation, we demonstrated gaping of the facets in the unstable segments. Two examples are shown below. In each case there was evidence of advanced disc degeneration as well as loose ligaments around a facet joint. In CT scans of patients with a history of chronic low back pain and suspicion of segmental instability we also found facet remodelling changes associated with the abnormal repositioning of the facets.

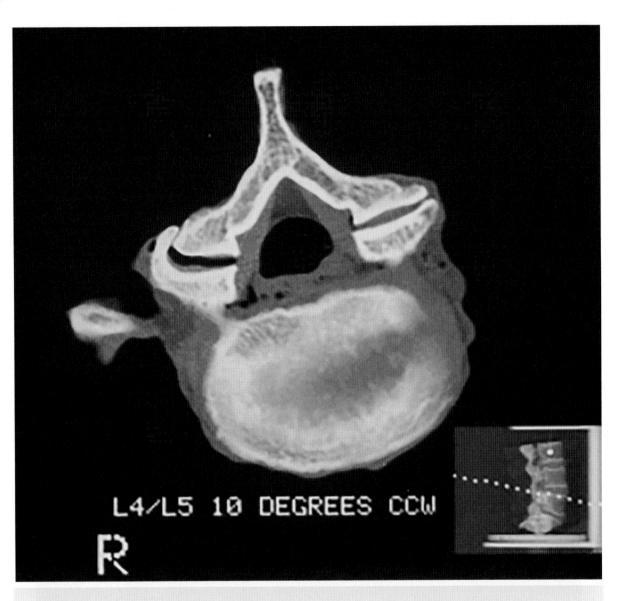

FIGURE 11.6 A CT image of a 57-year-old man with the spine in axial torsion

The gap opening up in the facet joint suggests loosening of ligaments in this motion segment. The affected segment shows a large osteophyte, suggestive of a previous injury.

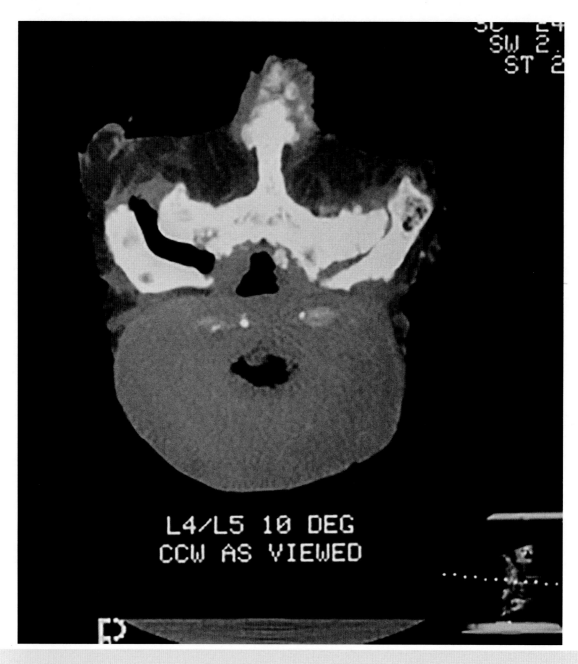

FIGURE 11.7 An axial view of facet gapping on torsion in an elderly cadaver lumbar motion segment from an 80-year-old man

Manual testing showed segmental instability.

Figures 11.6 and 11.7 are examples of L4 motion segments allowing abnormal axial rotation with gaping of the facet articular surfaces, as shown in CT of the fresh lumbar spine fixed in torsion (McFadden & Taylor, 1990).

This spine also shows vacuum phenomenon in the disc indicating disc degeneration.

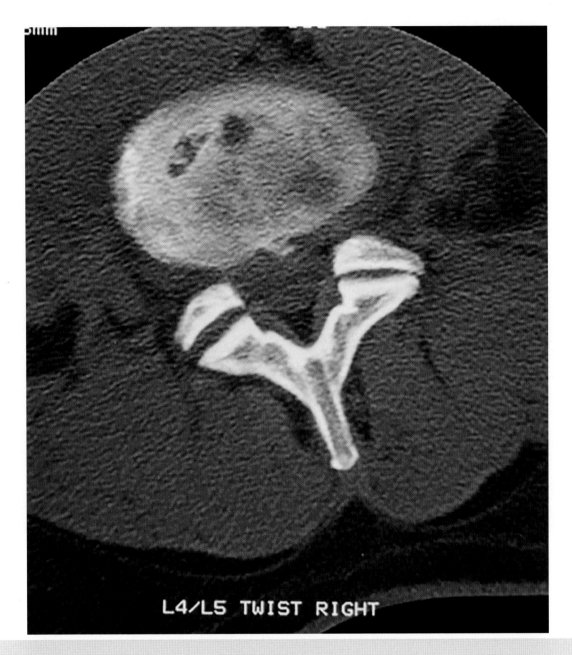

L4/L5 TWIST RIGHT

FIGURE 11.8 CT scan of an unstable segment, held in torsion, in a patient with clinical evidence of motion segment instability

Abnormal axial rotation in L4–5 with gaping of the facets in a patient with clinical instability.

Note the vacuum phenomenon in the degenerate disc.

Disc degeneration is witnessed by vacuum phenomenon. There is no gross distortion but there is facet separation in a 'loose joint' (Simon et al., 2012). As yet, there is no evidence of muscle atrophy.

Facet remodelling in unstable motion segments

In loose motion segments there are unilateral or bilateral changes in facet shape and position due to the repositioning of the facets with new bone or cartilage formation.

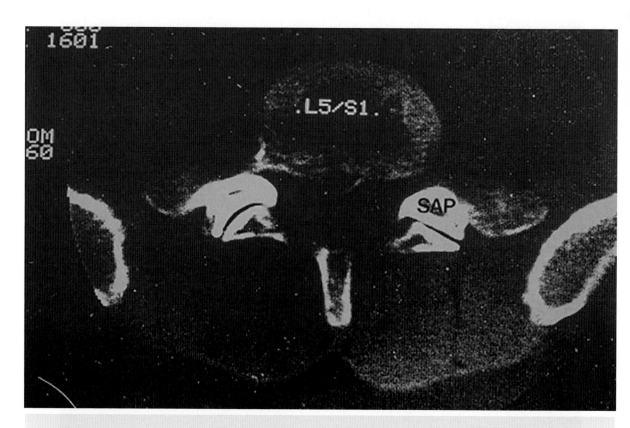

FIGURE 11.9 CT from a patient with chronic low back pain

The facets on the left are of normal shape and position, while those on the right are flattened, suggesting probable instability.

The flattened inferior articular process is subluxed backwards on the superior articular process (SAP). The ligamentum flavum grows backwards to fill the space.

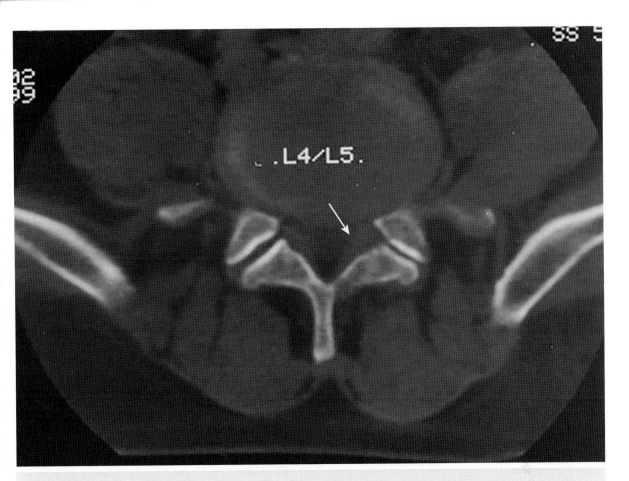

FIGURE 11.10 Subluxed inferior articular processes at L4–5 in a 48-year-old man with chronic back pain

There is rounding of posterior surfaces where new articular cartilage is formed due to pressure and movement on the thickened posterior capsule. The ligamentum flavum fills the gaps in front of the displaced inferior articular process (small arrow). The deep multifidus muscles show fatty atrophy.

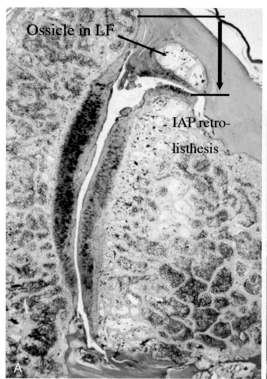

Ossicle in LF

IAP retro-
listhesis

A

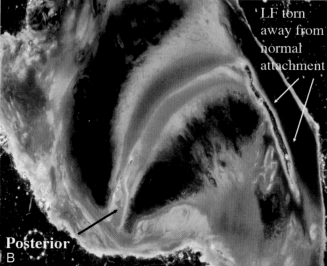

LF torn
away from
normal
attachment

Posterior

B

FIGURE 11.11 Capsular changes

A) The thick section on the right shows separation of the ligamentum flavum from its normal attachment to the inferior articular process (IAP).

B) The thin section on the left shows minor retrolisthesis of the inferior articular process with formation of a small ossicle in the ligamentum flavum (LF).

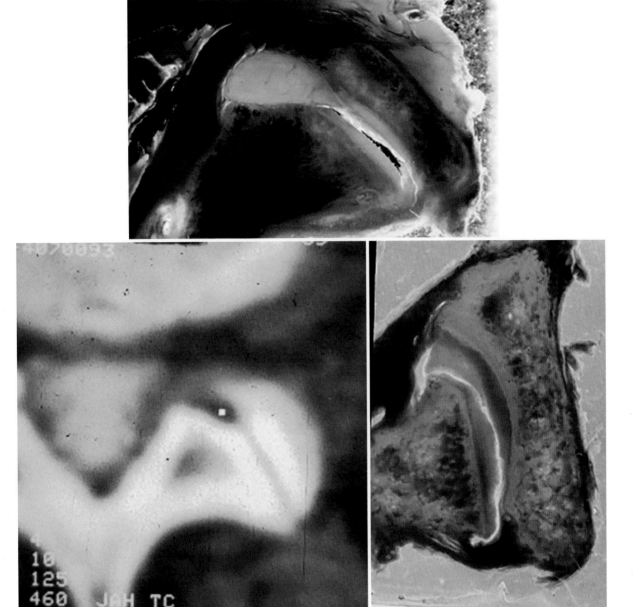

FIGURE 11.12 Enlarged fat pads at mid-joint level in thick sections from patients with back pain and probable segmental instability

The placement of the white dot allows measurement of tissue density to identify fat. Normally, the synovial-lined fat pads are confined to the polar recesses of lumbar facet (Taylor & McCormick, 1991) joints but in these 'loose joints' the fat pads enlarge and extend to mid-joint level, like padding to fill the void.

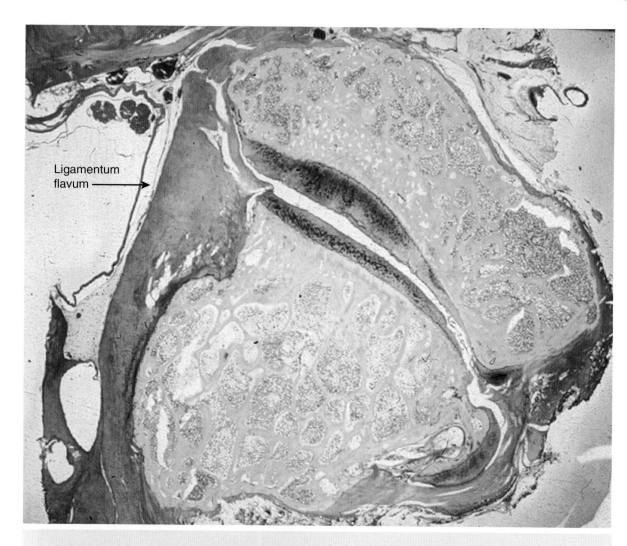

Ligamentum flavum

FIGURE 11.13 A 100-micron transverse section of a lower lumbar facet joint shows formation of new articular cartilage where retrolisthesis of the inferior articular process causes the 'loose' facet to rub on the thick posterior capsule

Posterior remodelling in a 'loose' joint: In this 100-micron section, new articular cartilage has formed on the superior articular process where it rubbed against the thickened posterior capsule. See also Figure 12.9.

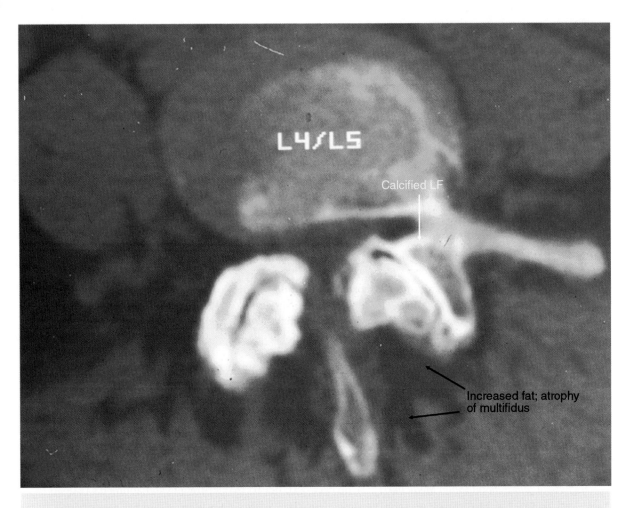

FIGURE 11.14 Formation of large marginal osteophytes around degenerate facet joints in a 'loose' motion segment

These may help to stabilise a segment, sometimes by fusion across the unstable segment.

Gross hypertrophy of arthritic facets or spontaneous inter-facet or interbody fusions may stabilise an unstable motion segment (LF = ligamentum flavum).

References

Beutler, WJ, Fredrickson, BE, Murtland, A et al. 2003 The natural history of spondylolysis and spondylolisthesis: 45-year follow-up evaluation. *Spine*, 28(10), pp. 1027–1035; discussion p. 1035. doi:10.1097/01.BRS.0000061992.98108.A0

Farfan, H 1973 *Mechanical disorders of the low back*. Lea and Febiger, Philadelphia.

Farfan, HF & Gracovetsky, S 1984 The nature of instability. *Spine*, 9(7), pp. 714–719. doi:10.1097/00007632-198410000-00011

Hardcastle, P, Annear, P, Foster, DH et al. 1992 Spinal abnormalities in young fast bowlers. *Journal of Bone & Joint Surgery, British*, 74(3), pp. 421–425. doi:10.1302/0301-620X.74B3.1587894

Kotilainen, E, Heinanen, J, Gullichsen, E et al. 1997 Spondylodesis in the treatment of segmental instability of the lumbar spine with special reference to clinically verified instability. *Acta Neurochirurgica (Wien)*, 139(7), pp. 629–635. doi:10.1007/BF01411998

Lehmann, TR & Brand, RA 1983 Instability of the lumbar spine. *Journal of Orthopaedic Translation*, 7(97), pp. 155–163.

McFadden, KD & Taylor, JR 1990 Axial rotation in the lumbar spine and gaping of the zygapophyseal joints. *Spine*, 15(4), pp. 295–299. doi:10.1097/00007632-199004000-00009

Ohmori, K, Ishida, Y, Takatsu, T et al. 1995 Vertebral slip in lumbar spondylolysis and spondylolisthesis. Long-term follow-up of 22 adult patients. *Journal of Bone & Joint Surgery, British*, 77(5), pp. 771–773.

O'Sullivan, PB, Phyty, GD, Twomey, LT & Allison, GT 1997 Evaluation of specific stabilizing exercise in the treatment of chronic low back pain with radiologic diagnosis of spondylolysis or spondylolisthesis. *Spine*, 22(24), pp. 2959–2967. doi:10.1097/00007632-199712150-00020

Schwarzer, AC, Aprill, CN, Derby, R et al. 1994 The relative contributions of the disc and zygapophyseal joint in chronic low back pain. *Spine*, 19(7), pp. 801–806. doi:10.1097/00007632-199404000-00013

Simon, P, Espinoza Orias, AA, Andersson, GB et al. 2012 In vivo topographic analysis of lumbar facet joint space width distribution in healthy and symptomatic subjects. *Spine*, 37(12), pp. 1058–1064. doi:10.1097/BRS.0b013e3182552ec9

Taylor, JR & McCormick, CC 1991 Lumbar facet joint fat pads: their normal anatomy and their appearance when enlarged. *Neuroradiology*, 33(1), pp. 38–42. doi:10.1007/BF00593331

Taylor, J, Twomey, L & Levander, B 2000 Contrasts between cervical and lumbar motion segments. *Critical Reviews in Physical and Rehabilitation Medicine*, 12(4), pp. 345–371. doi:10.1615/critrevphysrehabilmed.v12.i4.40

Taylor, M, Taylor, J & McCormick, C 1992 Features associated with subluxation of lumbar facet joints. Paper presented at the Society of Human Biology.

Teplick, JG, Laffey, PA, Berman, A & Haskin, ME 1986 Diagnosis and evaluation of spondylolisthesis and/or spondylolysis on axial CT. *American Journal of Neuroradiology*, 7(3), pp. 479–491.

Tokuhashi, Y, Matsuzaki, H & Sano, S. 1993 Evaluation of clinical lumbar instability using the treadmill. *Spine*, 18(15), pp. 2321–2324. doi:10.1097/00007632-199311000-00031

Wang, J & Yang, X 2009 Age-related changes in the orientation of lumbar facet joints. *Spine*, 34(17), pp. E596–598. doi:10.1097/BRS.0b013e3181abbf1e

Further reading

Kirkaldy-Willis, WH & Farfan, HF 1982 Instability of the lumbar spine. *Clinical Orthopaedics and Related Research*, (165), pp. 110–123.

CHAPTER 12

SPINAL STENOSIS

Arthritic changes and instability can both lead to narrowing of the space for spinal nerves in the spinal canal or the intervertebral foramen, with pressure on these nerves causing sciatica with both sensory and motor impairments. Prolonged pressure may cause permanent damage to the nerves with peripheral loss of sensation and motor function (Rydevik, Brown & Lundborg, 1984).

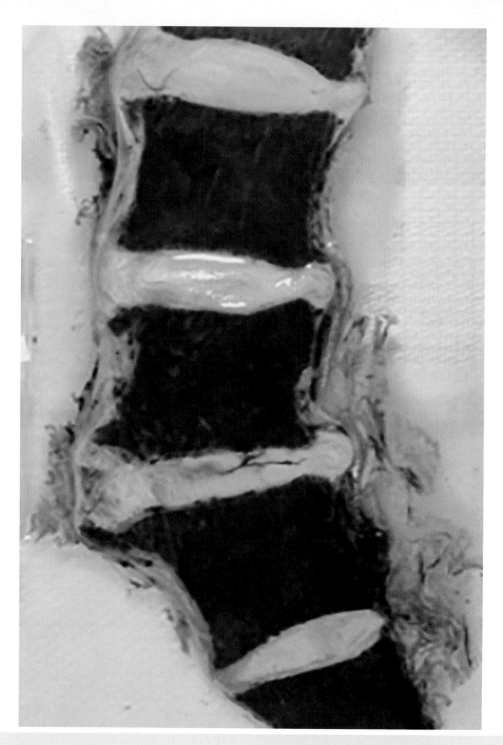

FIGURE 12.1 Spinal canal stenosis due to disc protrusion seen in thick sagittal section

The lumbo-sacral discs degenerate with fissures and disc protrusions.

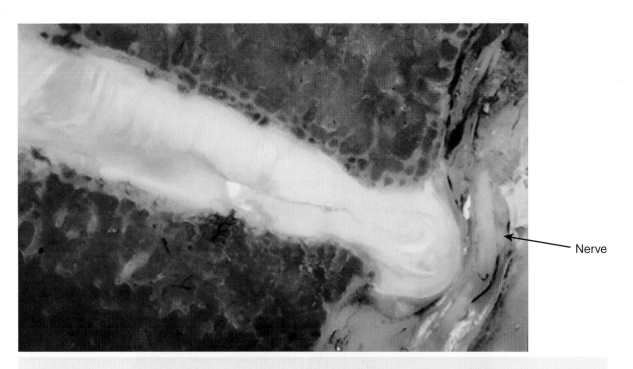

Nerve

FIGURE 12.2 A close view shows a spinal nerve pushed backwards by the disc prolapse into a confined space in the spinal canal

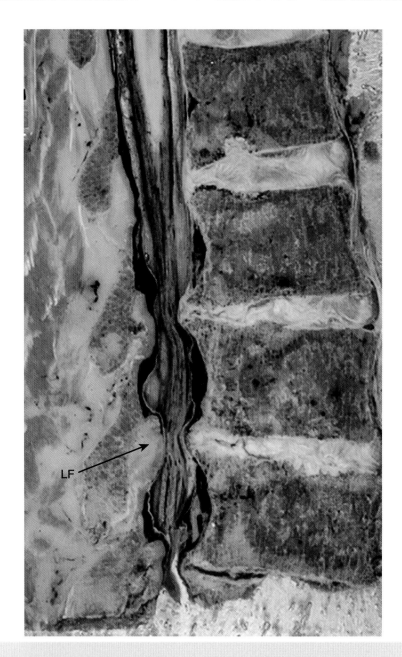

FIGURE 12.3 A thick sagittal section of L1–4 shows severe central stenosis in the spinal canal due to disc protrusions with marginal osteophytes

These impinge on the cauda equina from in front and bulging ligamenta flava (LF) press forwards at the same levels.

The lumbar discs are degenerate and fissured as seen in the sagittal sections of the lower vertebrae and the spinal canal. The normal conus of the spinal cord is seen at L1–2.

Compression of the cauda equina imperils their blood supply. Motor and sensory functions are impaired and could be permanently affected (Rydevik, Brown & Lundborg, 1984).

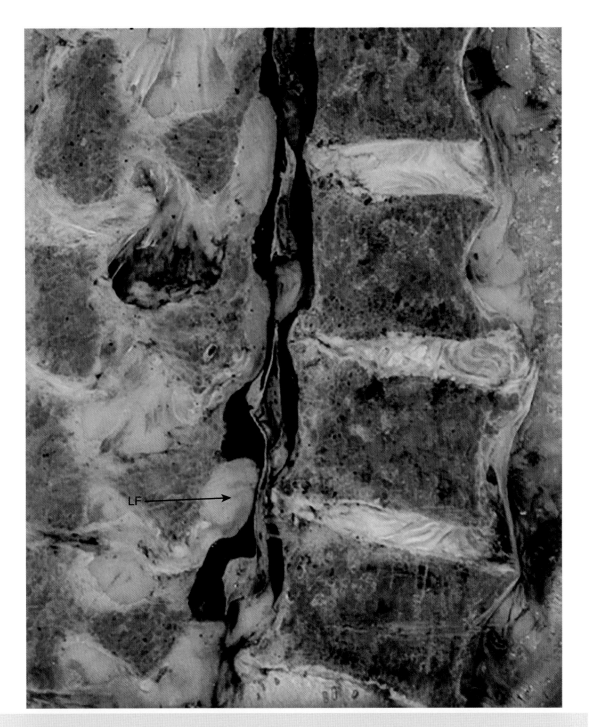

FIGURE 12.4 A thick parasagittal section shows lateral stenosis with encroachment on the lateral spinal canal by protruding discs and bulging ligamenta flava

The collapse of the discs allows swelling and bulging of the ligamenta flava.

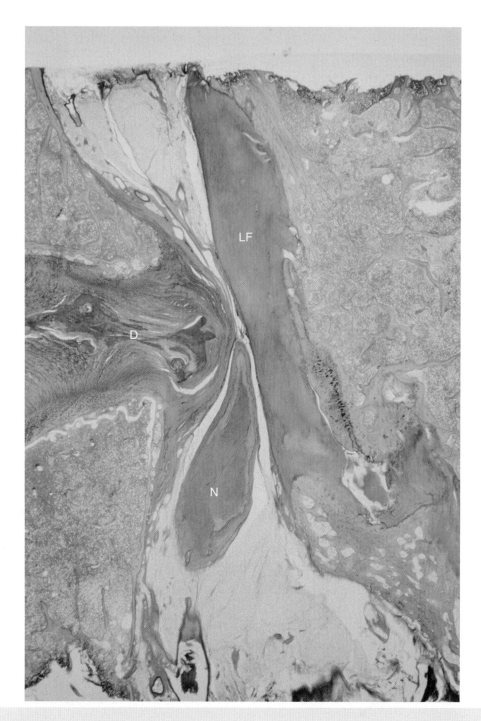

FIGURE 12.5 A stained 100-micron section shows stenosis of the lateral spinal canal due to disc herniation

A spinal nerve is compressed and deformed by the disc prolapse.

D: Disc, N: Nerve, LF: Ligamenta flava

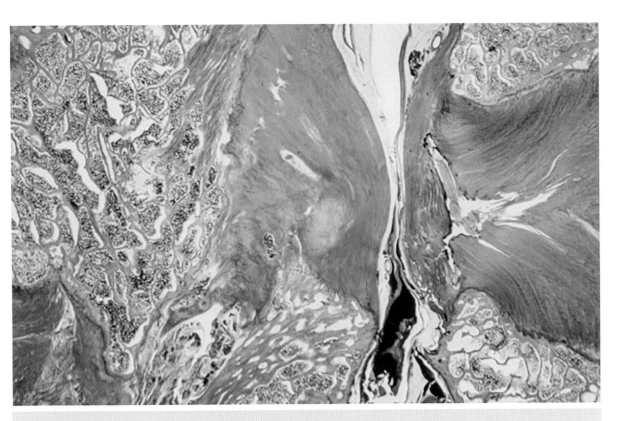

FIGURE 12.6 Disc degeneration and bulging forward of the ligamentum flavum compress a vein which contains a thrombus

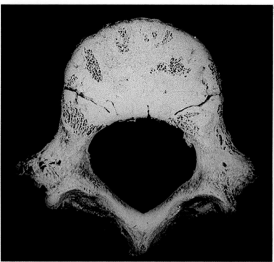 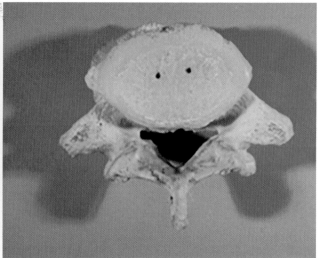

FIGURES 12.7 AND 12.8 The rounded shape of the spinal canal in youth (left) contrasts with the trefoil shape in old age (right)

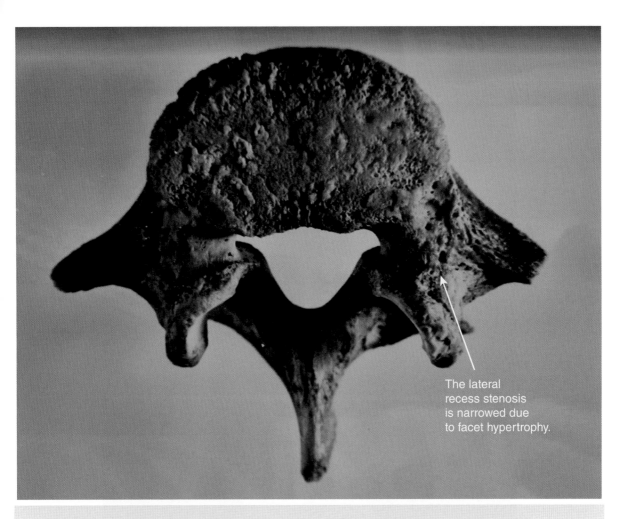

The lateral recess stenosis is narrowed due to facet hypertrophy.

FIGURE 12.9 Nerve root compression in the lateral recess

With ageing, hypertrophy of the facets may compress the spinal nerve in the foramen.

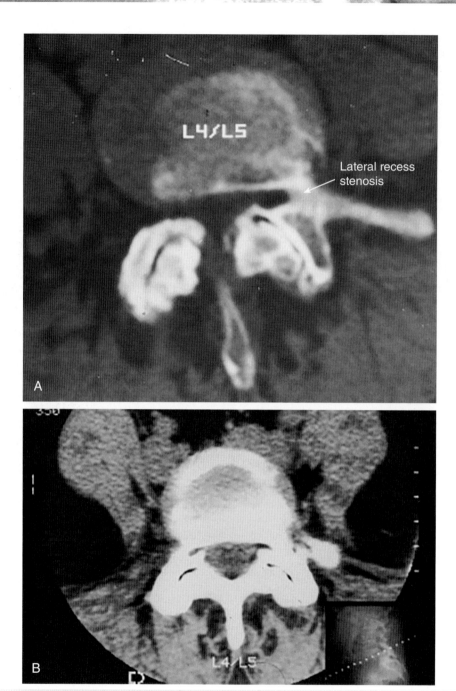

FIGURE 12.10 Examples of lateral recess stenosis in axial CT scans of elderly patients

A. Showing muscle wasting in multifidus (dark areas behind facets).

B. The nerve is constricted in the lateral recess between the posterior margin of the vertebral body and the anterior margin of the facet joint.

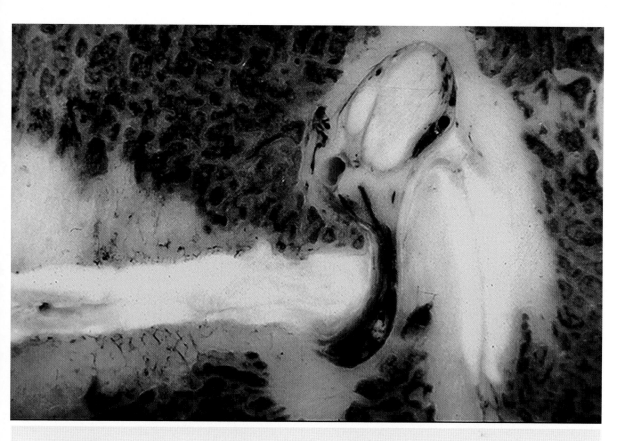

FIGURE 12.11 A thick sagittal section with accompanying diagram shows crowding of the nerve roots in foraminal stenosis due to loss of disc height

**Segmental instability
and foraminal stenosis**

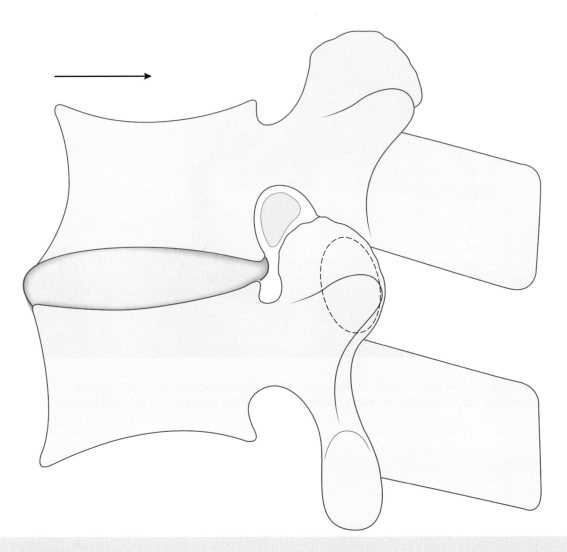

FIGURE 12.12

Diagram shows the nerve roots are crowded in the upper intervertebral foramen by facet hypertrophy and disc degeneration, which encroach on the space for the spinal nerves (Twomey & Taylor, 1988).

References

Rydevik, B, Brown, MD & Lundborg, G 1984 Pathoanatomy and pathophysiology of nerve root compression. *Spine*, 9(1), pp. 7–15. doi:10.1097/00007632-198401000-00004

Twomey, LT & Taylor, JR 1988 Age changes in the lumbar spine and intervertebral canals. *Paraplegia*, 26, pp. 238–249.

Further reading

Rawall, S, Mehndi, A & Nene, A 2010 Re: Janan Abbas, Kamal Hamoud, Masharawi YM, et al. Ligamentum flavum thickness in normal and stenotic lumbar spines. Spine 2010;35:1225-30. *Spine*, 35(26), pp. E1537–1538. doi:10.1097/BRS.0b013e318200c14a

CHAPTER 13

LUMBAR SPINAL INJURIES

The lumbar discs are vulnerable to rotational strain (Farfan et al., 1970), especially in flexion where the facets are only partly in contact, allowing greater torsion or translation so that they offer less protection against excessive strain in the disc. The lumbar vertebral bodies are vulnerable to flexion compression injuries causing multiple trabecular fractures with vertebral body collapse and bone bruising. This contrasts with the cervical spine where the injuries are more often at the linear disc/vertebral junction with annular tears at the vertebra rim, or more extensive linear separation of the disc from the vertebra.

Lumbar vertebral body injuries are more common than gross disc injuries. The acute injuries shown in this section are due to blunt trauma in a fall or a motor vehicle crash. Victims either died at the scene, most often from head injuries, or survived for a short period of days or weeks. The minor undisplaced facet injuries were not visible on post-mortem x-rays and were only demonstrated on sectioning (Taylor, Twomey & Corker, 1990; Taylor, Twomey & Levander, 2000).

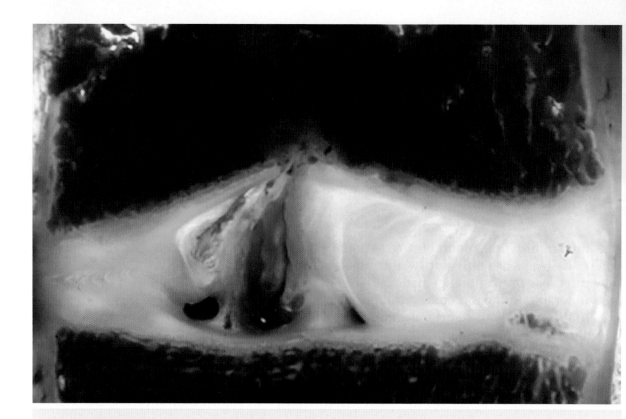

FIGURE 13.1 An acute injury shows a small central fracture of the vertebral endplate with bleeding into the nucleus pulposus below

Blood gives a high signal on MRI; bleeding into the disc may be demonstrable in acute injuries. A fractured endplate allows bleeding into the disc, and allows growth of blood vessels and nerves through the defect into the central disc, which is not normally innervated. This change provides another mechanism for onset of discogenic pain.

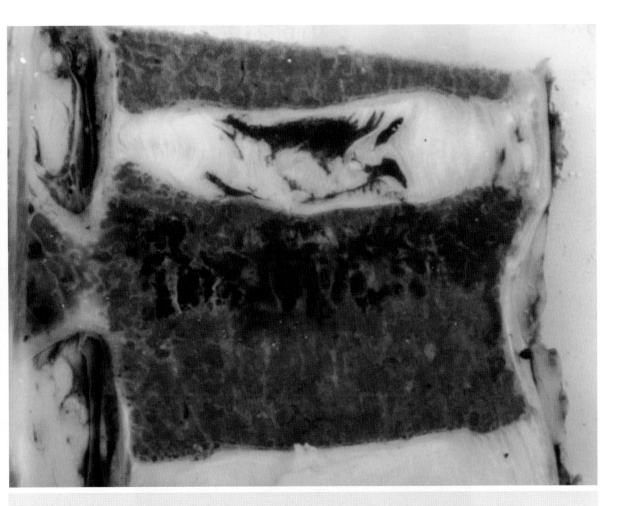

FIGURE 13.2 An axial compression injury of a vertebral body with multiple trabecular fractures

The thick sagittal section from a 49-year-old man shows widespread bone bruising with dark blood in the marrow spaces and bleeding into the central disc above, through an endplate fracture. The primary injury is to the vertebral body, with collapse of the vertebral endplate and bleeding into the nucleus pulposus above.

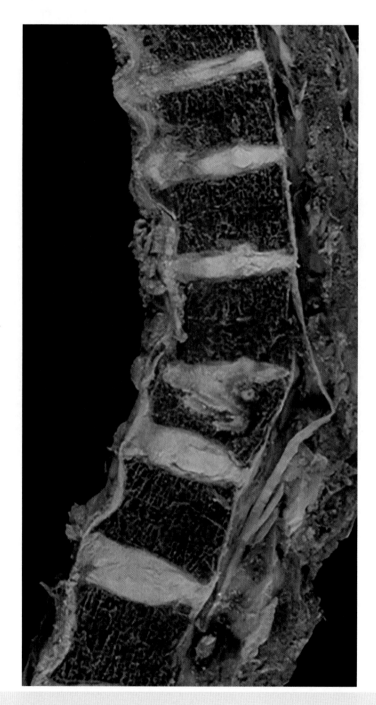

FIGURE 13.3 A sagittal section shows the long-term effects of a vertebral body crush fracture from flexion-compression

There is 'wedging' with loss of height anteriorly, laminar fusions behind and there may be narrowing of the spinal canal.

These are most common in the lower thoracic and upper lumbar vertebrae.

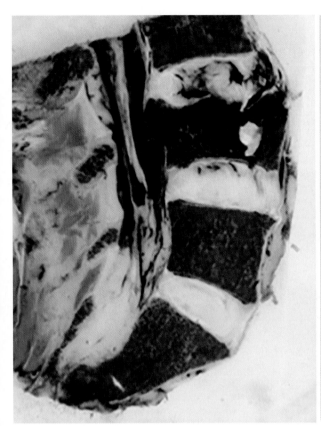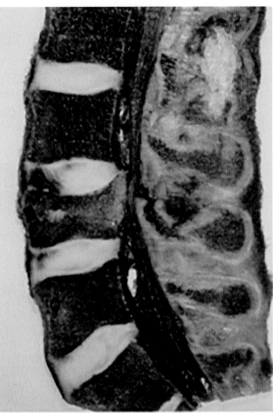

FIGURES 13.4 AND 13.5 Lower lumbar burst fractures: part of the vertebral body is displaced forwards and part moves backwards into the spinal canal

Left: A 49-year-old man crushed by a falling tree; Right: A pedestrian struck by a vehicle

In the example on the right (Figure 13.5) the spinal canal is occluded by the posterior fragment of the fractured L4 vertebral body, and the cauda equina are compressed.

DISC INJURIES

The outer annulus is vulnerable to over-stretch injury in hyperflexion or hyperextension. In erect posture, the facets are in full contact in the best position to resist translation and axial rotation; but in full flexion there is minimal articular contact and the spiral fibres of the annulus may be torn, especially in combined flexion and axial rotation.

Acute injuries to the outer annulus of the disc cause release of mediators of inflammation (Nygaard, Mellgren & Osterud, 1997).

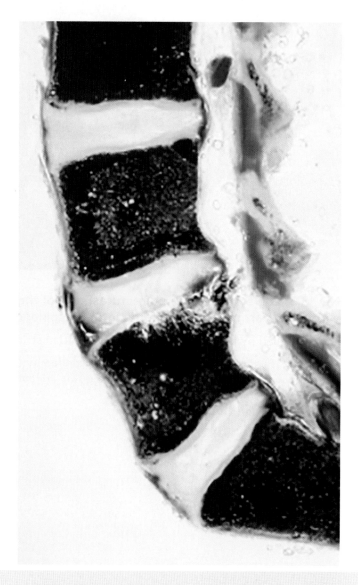

FIGURE 13.6 A thick sagittal section shows acute annulus injuries

There is bleeding in the anterior and posterior outer annulus in all discs, from hyperflexion and hyperextension stretch injuries of the collagenous lamellae.

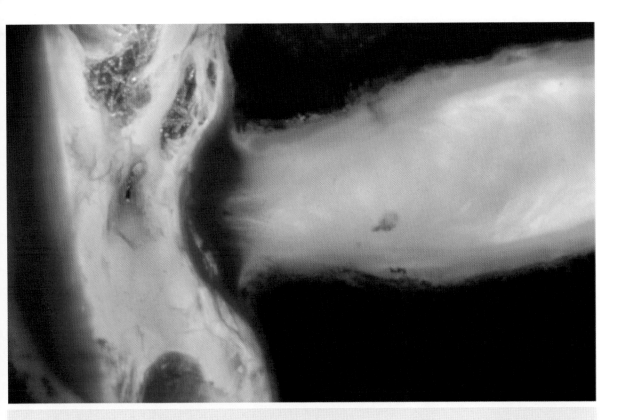

FIGURE 13.7   A closer view of L4–5 shows bleeding from the acute injuries into the postero-lateral outer annulus

The thick sagittal section (dark-ground illumination) shows acute injuries to the L4–5 posterior annulus fibrosus and also at the disc vertebral body junction wih bone bruising in the adjacent vertebral body. The outer annulus attaches to the vertebral rim so that flexion injury has affected both the annulus and posterior vertebral rim.

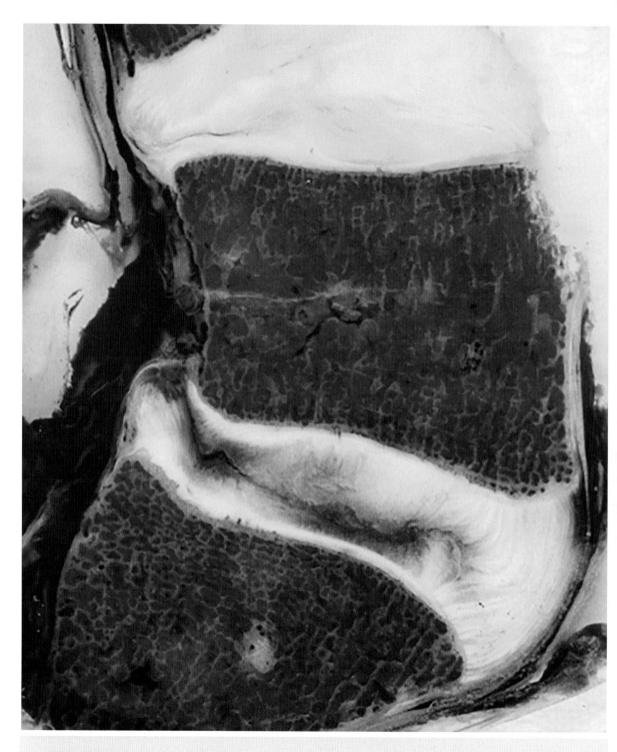

FIGURE 13.8 An isolated disc injury to L5–S1 in a 43-year-old man: The sagittal section shows blood staining around an extensive fissure

FACET INJURIES

The facet injuries described here were observed in spines that appeared to be free of fractures in their post-mortem x-rays. The blunt trauma facet injuries only became visible on sectioning.

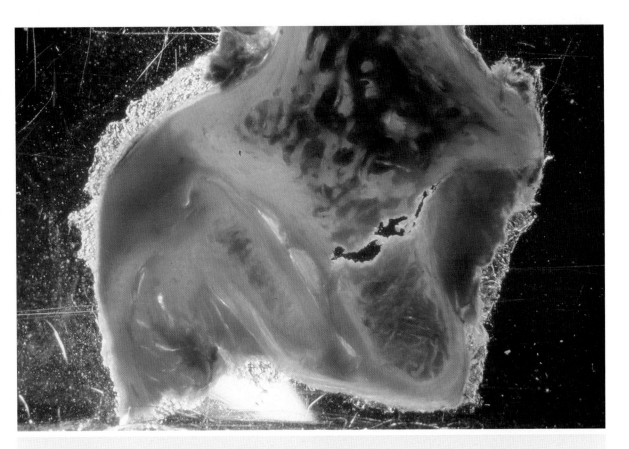

FIGURE 13.9 A postero-central fracture of the superior articular process in a thick transverse section from a 23-year-old woman (dark-ground illumination)

The small undisplaced fractures almost all involve the superior articular process.

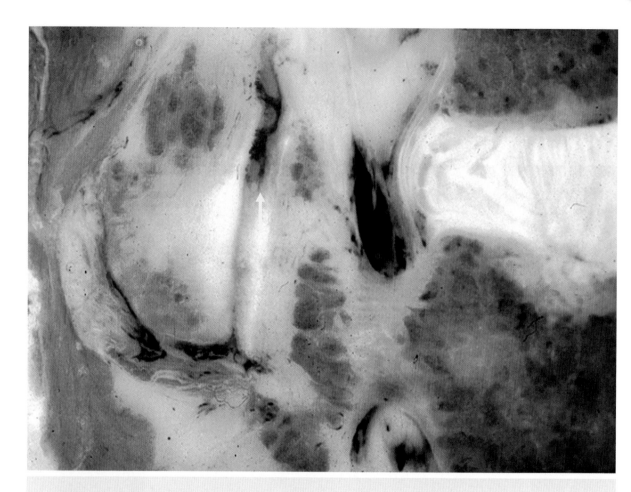

FIGURE 13.10 This minor articular injury, in a thick sagittal section, shows upper articular surface injury with haemarthrosis spreading to both upper and lower joint recesses

The injury to the upper joint surfaces appears to be confined to the articular cartilages.

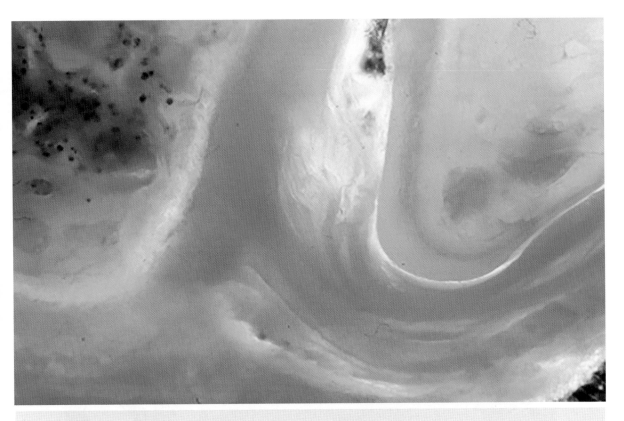

FIGURE 13.11 A capsular tear in a thick unstained sagittal section where the capsule attaches to the articular cartilage

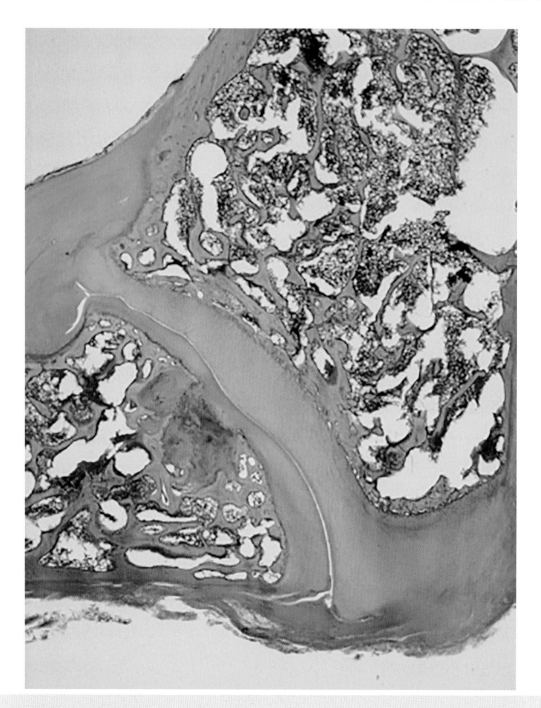

FIGURE 13.12 Transverse section (100-microns) of a lumbar facet joint in a child showing a small, healing, central facet fracture

This healing microfracture is seen in a lumbar inferior articular process of a child who survived a fall of five metres for three weeks but died of head injuries.

Note the deformation of the articular cartilage adjacent to the site of the fracture callus.

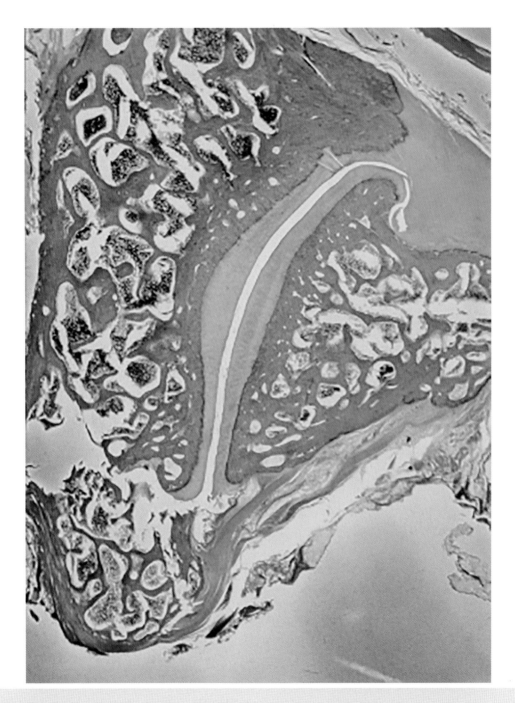

FIGURE 13.13 A fracture of a mamillary process in a 19-year-old man in a 100-micron stained transverse section

The facet fracture observed here is suggestive of the mamillary process being pulled off the superior articular process by tension in the attachment of multifidus combined with the forward impact to the concave superior articular process by the convex inferior articular process.

References

Farfan, HF, Cossette, JW, Robertson, GH et al.1970 The effects of torsion on the lumbar intervertebral joints: the role of torsion in the production of disc degeneration. *Journal of Bone & Joint Surgery, American*, 52(3), pp. 468–497.

Nygaard, OP, Mellgren, SI & Osterud, B 1997 The inflammatory properties of contained and noncontained lumbar disc herniation. *Spine*, 22(21), pp. 2484–2488. doi:10.1097/00007632-199711010-00004

Taylor, JR, Twomey, LT & Corker, M 1990 Bone and soft tissue injuries in post-mortem lumbar spines. *Paraplegia*, 28(2), pp. 119–129. doi:10.1038/sc.1990.14

Taylor, J, Twomey, L & Levander, B 2000 Contrasts between cervical and lumbar motion segments. *Critical Reviews in Physical and Rehabilitation Medicine*, 12(4), pp. 345–371. doi:10.1615/critrevphysrehabilmed.v12.i4.40

CHAPTER 14

LUMBAR METASTASES

In our survey of a large number of spines, we encountered cases of metastatic tumours in lumbar vertebral bodies. It is important in unexplained onset of low back pain to consider the possibility of lumbar spinal metastases. Examples are shown.

The valveless veins of the epidural plexus (see Figure 6.2) allow movement of tumour cells from viscera into the spine.

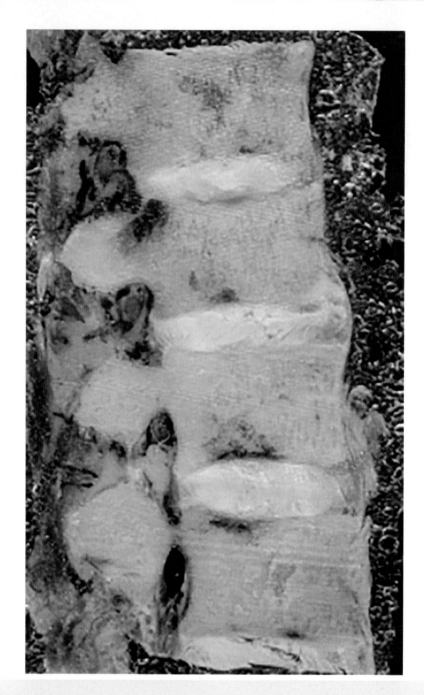

FIGURE 14.1 Prostatic metastases throughout all the vertebral bodies with reactive sclerosis

Reactive sclerosis makes the vertebral bodies pale in colour.

Invasion of the vertebral arch is a late phenomenon. The vertebral bodies show reactive changes to the presence of tumour cells. The discs are not invaded though there are reactive vascular changes at the disc vertebral junctions.

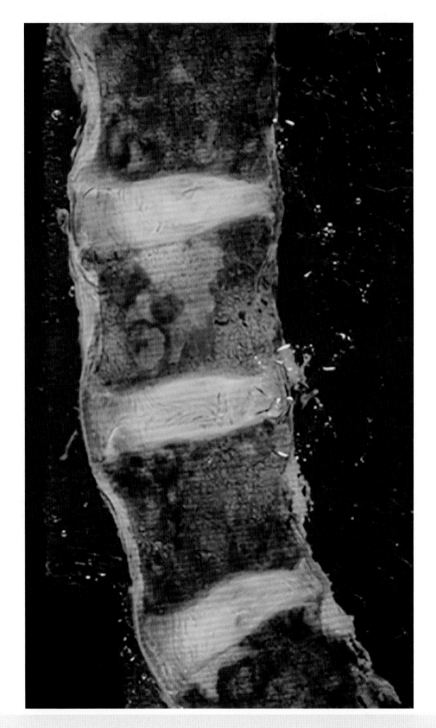

FIGURE 14.2 A thick sagittal section shows scattered metastases in lumbar vertebrae

Ovarian metastases replacing normal bone in vertebral bodies. Once again, the discs are not invaded.

LUMBAR PATHOLOGY AND LOW BACK PAIN

We have not dealt systematically with the topic of low back pain, but we have described lesions causing acute pain from injury and lesions associated with chronic low back pain or sciatica. We have described the anatomical basis for discogenic and facet pain (Schwarzer et al., 1994), and we have outlined the segmental distribution of dermatomes and myotomes which may be affected by sciatica in age spinal stenosis.

Reference

Schwarzer, AC, Aprill, CN, Derby, R et al. 1994 The relative contributions of the disc and zygapophyseal joint in chronic low back pain. *Spine*, 19(7), pp. 801–806. doi:10.1097/00007632-199404000-00013

Further reading

Bogduk, N & Long, DM 1979 The anatomy of the so-called 'articular nerves' and their relationship to facet denervation in the treatment of low-back pain. *Journal of Neurosurgery*, 51(2), pp. 172–177. doi:10.3171/jns.1979.51.2.0172

Butt, AM, Gill, C, Demerdash, A et al. 2015 A comprehensive review of the sub-axial ligaments of the vertebral column: part I anatomy and function. *Child's Nervous System*, 31(7), pp. 1037–1059. doi:10.1007/s00381-015-2729-z

Moore, RJ, Osti, OL, Vernon-Roberts, B & Fraser, RD 1992 Changes in endplate vascularity after an outer anulus tear in the sheep. *Spine*, 17(8), pp. 874–878. doi:10.1097/00007632-199208000-00003

Peng, B, Wu, W, Hou, S et al. 2005 The pathogenesis of discogenic low back pain. *Journal of Bone & Joint Surgery, British*, 87(1), pp. 62–67.

Schwarzer, AC, Aprill, CN, Derby, R et al. 1995 The prevalence and clinical features of internal disc disruption in patients with chronic low back pain. *Spine*, 20(17), pp. 1878–1883. doi:10.1097/00007632-199509000-00007

Twomey, LT & Taylor, JR 1987 Age changes in lumbar vertebrae and intervertebral discs. *Clinical Orthopaedics and Related Research*, (224), pp. 97–104.

Varlotta, GP, Lefkowitz, TR, Schweitzer, M et al. 2011 The lumbar facet joint: a review of current knowledge: part 1: anatomy, biomechanics, and grading. *Skeletal Radiology*, 40(1), pp. 13–23. doi:10.1007/s00256-010-0983-4

Wilke, HJ, Zanker, D & Wolfram, U 2012 Internal morphology of human facet joints: comparing cervical and lumbar spine with regard to age, gender and the vertebral core. *Journal of Anatomy*, 220(3), pp. 233–241. doi:10.1111/j.1469-7580.2011.01465.x

BIBLIOGRAPHY

Giles, LG 1987 *The anatomy of lower lumbar and lumbosacral joint recesses with particular reference to their innervation.* University of Western Australia, Perth.

McFadden, KD & Taylor, JR 1990 Axial rotation in the lumbar spine and gaping of the zygapophyseal joints. *Spine*, 15(4), pp. 295–299.

Taylor, J 1974 *Growth and development of human intervertebral discs.* Edinburgh University, Edinburgh.

Taylor, JR 1975 Growth of human intervertebral discs and vertebral bodies. *Journal of Anatomy*, 120(Pt 1), pp. 49–68.

Taylor, J & Twomey, L 1980 Sagittal and horizontal plane movement of the human lumbar vertebral column in cadavers and in the living. *Rheumatology*, 19(4), pp. 223–232.

Taylor, JR & Twomey, LT 1986 Age changes in lumbar zygapophyseal joints: Observations on structure and function. *Spine*, 11(7), pp. 739–745.

Taylor, J, Twomey, L & Levander, B 2000 Contrasts between cervical and lumbar motion segments. *Critical Reviews in Physical and Rehabilitation Medicine*, 12(4), pp. 345–371.

Twomey, LT 1981 *Age changes in the human lumber vertebral column.* University of Western Australia, Perth.

Twomey, L & Taylor, J 1982 Flexion creep deformation and hysteresis in the lumbar vertebral column. *Spine*, 7(2), pp. 116–122.

INDEX

Page numbers followed by "*f*" or "*t*" indicate figures or tables.